The Pizza and Ice Cream Diet

The Pizza and Ice Cream Diet

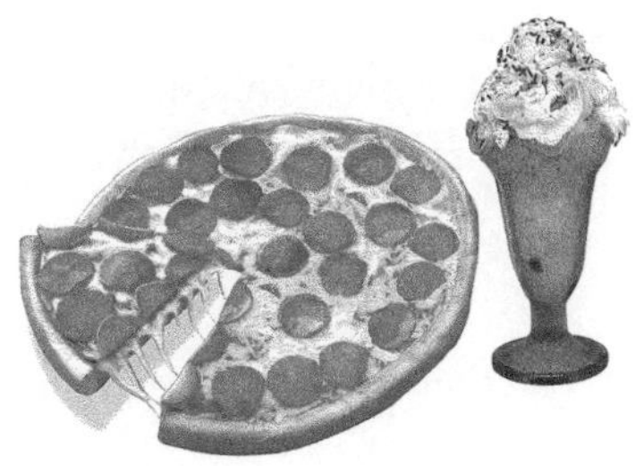

Barbara Tessari

Jodomi Books

The Pizza and Ice Cream Diet

Jodomi Books

http://www.pizzaandicecreamdiet.com

Manufactured in the United States of America
Library of Congress Catalog Number: 2002090463
ISBN 0-9718036-0-9

Cover Design: JOW Graphics
Page Design: Antoinette D'Amore
Editorial Assistance: Charles Wetherall and Christine LePorte

Library of Congress Cataloging-in-Publication Data
Tessari, Barbara Ryan (Barbara Ryan Tessari)
Jodomi Books
The Pizza And Ice Cream Diet

1. Diet 2. Weight Loss 3. Behavior Change I. Title

When I said I needed to get a real job, she said I was a writer. When I asked, "What do I know?" she said, "Sounds like you know a lot." When I said I was wasting my time she said finishing this book was one of the most important things I could do for myself. She was right. Thank you, Melissa.

Contents

Acknowledgements

Writing the words was easy. Making the words a book was the hardest thing I have ever done.

Writing is a lonely business and without the support and help of others, one would go mad.

Instrumental to my accomplishment were the people in my life who helped me, not only with the actual production of this book, but also with their unending support – each offered in their own unique way.

To Chuck, who was always there for me when I needed a question answered, or an honest opinion, and lifted me up when I was down. He allowed me to believe I could finish this book and was worthy of that right.

To Joann, whose delicious cover design turned my muddied fantasy into a visual reality. And to Antoinette, who creatively displayed my words.

To Sandy, who's *always* there for me.

To my kids, who put up with me constantly shooing them away. I regret I will never get back that time with them – a price I had to pay.

And especially to my husband, who constantly told me, "Just finish the darn thing."

Preface

About two years ago, I was channel surfing. I listened to seven infomercials making ridiculous claims about a new diet, pill or exercise machine. Channel by channel – one after the other – they came. "Get the body you always dreamed of in 15 minutes a day!" "Melt fat while you sleep!" "Eat all the foods you want and still lose weight!" I could feel the heat rising within me.

"Without *dangerous* exercise – guaranteed!" one boasted.

"That's it!" I exploded. "I can't take it anymore! I can't believe people are still believing and buying this nonsense!" Something had to be done. The madness had to stop. And so my journey began.

I agonized over what to say. What was my point? Does anyone even care? Once I started venting my anger on paper, I realized I had a lot to say and a lot of people *did* care.

I wanted to reach out to everyone like me and help them make sense of the hundreds of different reasons we eat the way we do, exercise the way we don't and generally feel lousy about ourselves.

Everyone can relate. Well, almost everyone. After all, there are a lucky small percentage of us who don't have a weight or food issue. But then again, they wouldn't pick up this book in the first place. The sad fact is that most of us do have at least a small problem with food. And if you picked up this book, then you do too.

I spent two years writing this book, but I spent 30 years doing research. My *life* was my research for I was a victim too. I spent my life learning, refining, obsessing, succeeding, failing and finally overcoming not just my weight problem, but also my food obsession.

As the book evolved, I learned a lot from my conversations with people about how they eat, why they eat and how they feel about themselves. Not only did I find that many people shared my torturous experiences with food, I discovered other attitudes and conclusions I had not recognized.

Today's distorted image of the "ideal" body and the confusion and misrepresentation of nutrition information have only added to our problem. We choose food over health, and we choose looks over health. We think we'd be better, happier, and more deeply loved, if only we could lose our extra weight.

That goal, as you know, is getting harder to achieve. Some of us are obsessed with the goal. Some just don't care any more. Not only are we giving up on our bodies, we are giving up on *ourselves*.

Health professionals and the media are coming to one conclusion about the adverse physical, and most importantly, *psychological* effects of dieting. *Diets don't work.* The diet industry phenomenon has reached its peak and we are finally recognizing its adverse effects. It's now up to us to reverse the damage it has done to our waistline, our relationship with food and ourselves.

But reversing the damage is easier said than done. After a long and arduous struggle, I've freed myself from my food and weight obsession. I've never felt better about myself. I've never been happier. Now, I want to help others set themselves free too.

But, how do I reach out to people who have unsuccessfully tried to lose weight again and again? How can I give them the power to change? How can I relate to the size 4 who's obsessed with a little cellulite and the 350-pound woman who's in denial and depression? How can I relate to the person who only wants to lose 10 pounds? How do I talk about nutrition when some people eat healthy and some consider the lettuce and tomato on their Whopper as their vegetable quota for the day. What about the person who craves sugar versus the person who craves fat; the person whose weight problem is a symptom of low self-esteem and the person who only has "some bad eating habits."

The truth is, I don't have the answer to the problem. You know why? We all don't have the same problem. Psychologically, a bulimic weighing 96 pounds may have issues similar to an emotional eater weighing 250 pounds; while two people who need to lose 30 pounds can have completely different reasons why they are overweight.

I can't give you *the* answer. But I can help you find *your* answer.

When you read this book, you may say from time to time, "I don't have that problem." That's okay. I know that. That's the point. Our weight issues are unique. But you may find reasons for your problem you hadn't previously realized. You may learn about the problems of others and thereby get a better understanding of your own.

I have put myself at risk by revealing secrets about myself that were never known to others. I felt it was important to share my secret thoughts, feelings and actions with regard to food and my perception of myself in order to help others. My words I share with you, while based on applied knowledge, come from the heart. Your challenge is to find yourself within these pages. Maybe you will find secrets that you've been hiding from yourself. Once you recognize the real reason you picked up this book, you can decide what you want to do about it. We all have *different* issues regarding our weight, our relationship with food and the perception of ourselves.

The only one who can find the answer is you.

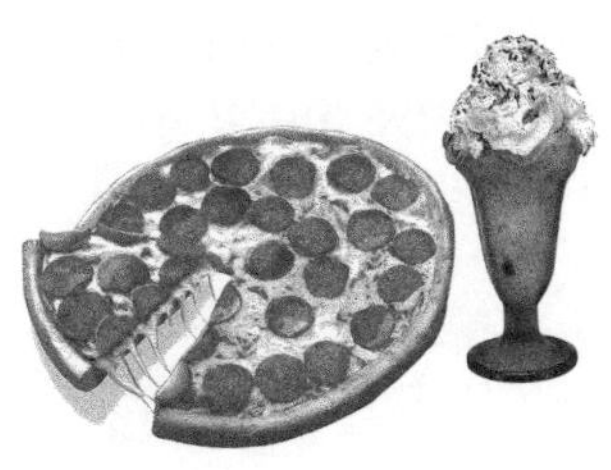

Chapter 1

The Pizza and Ice Cream Diet

You probably picked up this book thinking, "Wow! I can eat pizza and ice cream and still lose weight?" You plunked down your money and anxiously raced ahead to find the "magic."

Sorry to say, but just like other popular diet books, you'll find there is no "magic." *The Pizza and Ice Cream Diet* is not a miracle diet that claims you can gorge on foods like pizza and ice cream – and lose weight. On the other hand, it doesn't condemn such a diet either. The reality is you can lose weight by eating pizza and ice cream and most of us who are successful at losing weight do follow *The Pizza and Ice Cream Diet.*

Ironically, most of us insist on following any diet ***but*** *The Pizza and Ice Cream Diet.* We prefer to believe illogical, unproven food theories and so we buy, try and then fail each and every one of them. And sometimes we fail at the same diet over and over again. It seems the more we find new ways to lose weight, the fatter we become.

Meanwhile, our society has made the goal of being thin even harder to achieve. We've defined the ideal body as an unrealistic fantasy achievable only by a select few "aesthetically gifted" individuals. The diet industry claims obtaining the coveted look is not only easy, but success is guaranteed in six weeks. Food marketers lure us into eating foods that are convenient, fattening and nearly void of nutritional value. And to make the problem worse, our lifestyles have allowed moving our body to be optional.

The result? Now our minds – not our bodies – are dictating what foods we want and how much we want. We treat exercise like it's a form of punishment instead of something fun and we have become so critical and self-conscious about our bodies it's invading how we feel about ourselves. Failure, confusion and hopelessness have been the result of this decade of diet disillusionment.

It's time to get back to reality. It's time to start over in a new – and better – direction. The answer is not in another diet, product or pill. The "real" magic lies within you. *The Pizza and Ice Cream Diet* can help you find it.

Dieting Equals Failure

While you can lose weight using fad diets, the failure rate can be as high as 95 percent, according to the Federal Food and Drug Administration. *Ninety-five percent!* That means by spending money on these theories and products your chances of losing weight successfully are a measly five percent.

But millions of people have successfully lost weight and, more importantly, keep it off. So how did they do it? How did I do it? What's our secret? How can you do it?

What's This Book About?

The Pizza and Ice Cream Diet reveals the truth behind some of the more popular diets, gimmicks and gadgets that we've spent billions of dollars on in recent years. It reveals why they work or why they fail.

The book exposes the luring but deceptive marketing strategies of food manufacturers to sell products under the guise of being "healthy." It seems the more we know, the less we know. The situation has left us in a state of confusion. We don't know what to eat anymore.

Rather than give you more confusing information, this book will unravel the confusion and teach you how to be a better "consumer" of food.

It's an analysis of our obsession with food, our bodies, how we value ourselves and how we got that way in the first place. The process gives you the tools you need in order to change and *then* teaches you what to change to achieve realistic, lifetime results.

The book is an autobiography of sorts with my struggles and triumphs with food looking back on 30 years of grueling experience. I spent most of my life obsessing over food and exercise in pursuit of the perfect body. I used the mirror and a dress size to validate my self-worth.

After 30 years of self-abuse caused by my irrational view of food and a distorted perception of myself I finally recognized the destruction and decided to put an end to it. I came to terms with it all, took a new direction and started over. That's when I realized I had the secret to permanent weight loss all along. I realized I had the power not only to keep my weight off, but also to feel better about myself for who I was, not what I thought I was or obsessed to be. I want to share my secret with you.

What's Different About This Book?

The "magic" to The Pizza and Ice Cream Diet is the path it takes to finding your answer. When I discovered my answer, I recognized that the solution to my problems had not been delivered in the hundreds of diet books published today.

Some books do provide answers, but they aren't delivering all the information needed to succeed. We buy a self-help book that explores why we eat; we buy a nutrition book that tells us what to eat. And when we can't find the answer, or don't want to accept the answer, we rely on diet books that promise the easy answer – only it never delivers.

The reality is for most of us it's a combination of issues. And in today's environment, there are even more issues to address – some you might not even recognize. If you have more than one problem, you can't solve all your problems with one answer. It's like a puzzle. If there are missing pieces, you can't finish the puzzle.

The Pizza and Ice Cream Diet addresses all the issues. It follows a path to self-discovery.

Exploring the Real Issues

The Pizza and Ice Cream Diet explores the questions that *really* need to be answered. We don't need another way to lose weight; we need to know why we aren't losing weight. Why do I eat so much? Why can't I stop? Am I a carbohydrate addict? Am

I a food addict? What should I eat? Why do I hate myself for being fat? Why can't I be like her? Why can't I look like her? Why do I keep failing at diets? Is it my fault I'm fat?

The more we hear about food, the less educated and more obsessed we've become. Instead of overanalyzing what we eat, we should spend more time evaluating how we eat and why we eat. The reality is even if you have a personal nutrition chef and a drill sergeant for a trainer, if you're not mentally ready to lose weight, they may find you hiding in the closet having an affair with a box of Yodels at 2 a.m.

Humans come in different sizes and shapes. We all can't physically look alike no matter how hard we try. We are all unique. God made us that way. Just like no two fingerprints are alike, no two bodies are alike.

Most of us have weight issues. I don't say weight "problem" because many of us don't have a weight "problem" but we do have issues with our body and unmercifully define ourselves according to some misshapen idea about what we ought to look like.

Above All, Be Thin

We are becoming a society so obsessed with weight and the perfect body that even the most self-assured individuals are taking a second look at themselves and feeling ashamed of their bodies. Many of us seem to feel inferior, to some degree, to those who are fit, trim and especially those who work hard at achieving that coveted look. Imagine! A size 14 female surgeon or top executive might feel inferior to a size 4 sculpted personal trainer who barely graduated high school. Obviously, they are smart enough to know better, but trim figures in our society seem to be valued above everything.

Changing the Objective

Yet, there are still some people who are completely satisfied with themselves. What is their secret? You know whom I'm talking about. Not the ones spending countless hours in the gym and drinking protein shakes. I'm talking about the people who, when you mention Dr. Atkins, respond Dr. Who? They don't own a scale and only get weighed at their annual physical. They don't have gorgeous bodies but they aren't fat and they really don't seem to care that someone else's body might look better than theirs. We conclude they must have fast metabolisms and it has nothing to do with what they eat or don't eat. We say, "I'm not like them." We look for someone or something to blame for our eating problems. I used to think I was not like them too.

What if we all tried to be more like the satisfied people mentioned and less like an underwear model? Maybe if we stopped following diets and believing in hyped-up exercise commercials and accepted the fact that we aren't going to have the body we always wanted, maybe then we could be happy having a healthy mediocre body and get on with our lives.

Avoiding the Reality

We see weight loss as an insurmountable mountain to climb. Diet books rely on our desperation to sell substitutions for willpower and counting calories. The diet industry has profited immensely by selling unproven theories and formulas that "guarantee" to unlock the mystery of weight loss. We keep spending, trying and failing rather than face reality. Meanwhile the diet industry keeps reaping in the profits. And it seems to work no matter how bizarre the claim.

The truth is, any *real* success story comes from people who have enough willpower to give up some aspect of their present eating habits and lifestyle. They lose the weight primarily because they are eating fewer calories, not particular foods.

No Easy Way Out

You get up in the morning one day, look in the mirror and say, "Gee, I need to lose weight." And you want to lose the 20 pounds you gained over the last two years in two weeks! Cutting calories, using willpower, exercising, there's got to be an easier way. Well, there isn't! Wake up and smell the donuts!

I know I'm not telling you what you want to hear but don't get discouraged. Just think about it. If 95 percent of people who try all the miracle solutions fail, then maybe their solutions are harder to follow than the old way of losing weight motivated by the goal of just becoming "healthy."

The weight loss industry has caused us more harm than good. It has left us feeling inferior because we have even higher expectations of ourselves. The result? We are having more failures and more confusion. It has left us fat, broke and depressed.

Rome Wasn't Built . . .

We try to climb the mountain when we can't even get up the hill. But we don't want to climb the hill. We want weight loss to magically happen – today. We don't try to learn anything – we don't *want* to learn anything. Methods, theories, gadgets, pills and diets all promise to give us results and we can do it in 30 days. And when we don't see fast results, we say, "It didn't work." We quit until we find a new "magic" way to lose weight.

So why *aren't* we losing weight? Why are most of us still getting fatter? By all rights, we've spent enough money and there are enough information and products out there no one should be overweight! So what's the answer?

Find Your Problem

While there is no miracle answer to our failures, we can pinpoint a lot of the problems. But we can't just push a button and have a solution.

If you want to really get serious about changing the way you look, you've got to spend more time examining your *head*, not your diet. Not to say your diet doesn't have a lot to do with how much you weigh. It does.

But people who are successful at losing weight long term don't solve their problem by going on a diet. They do so because they are mentally ready to make a change. They identify their problem and make positive changes in their life to overcome their problem.

For most of us the problem isn't simple and it usually isn't just one problem. You may be in pain about other things besides your weight. You may have just picked up bad eating habits or have focused on food so much that you've become obsessed. Most likely it's a combination of habits, feelings and weaknesses that prevent you from succeeding. For now, it's time to forget about how much weight you need to lose.

Where to Start

The first step is to identify the problem. Most weight loss methods focus on what you eat or how you exercise. If followed, the diet or method may work; the gadget will give you results. Sadly, most of the methods fail because *we don't do them consistently.*

So if we know how, then why don't we *just do it!* And if our problem is we *won't do it* then how can we get ourselves *to do it!*

Finding Our Own Solutions

Even if you figure out why you don't do it, the reason you don't do it is probably different from the next person's. So maybe we should step back and take a look at ourselves and how, when and why we eat so we can find our own solutions to our problems.

I have many issues of my own. Much of what I have learned and now share with you comes from my own experiences. I don't have all the answers to your problems and the answers that worked for me may not work for you. But talking about my journey's successes, failures and personal conclusions have helped others find their answer. This book might help you find *your* answer too.

The Only Solution That Delivers

There is not much in this book that would be disputed by the experts. After years of trying to find a "magic" solution to my problem, I've finally realized that the majority of health professionals were right all along. They are the ones delivering the only "guaranteed" solution to our problems.

But the method we use to lose weight is only a small part of the solution. The real problem is our inability to want, accept and be empowered to change. Diets are only a Band-aid for the problem.

The path to get there is yours. Face reality, change your focus and get educated. Practice self-discovery in how you live your life and how you feel about yourself and food. *The Pizza and Ice Cream Diet* will help you get there. Find your own personal epiphany and you will never have to diet again.

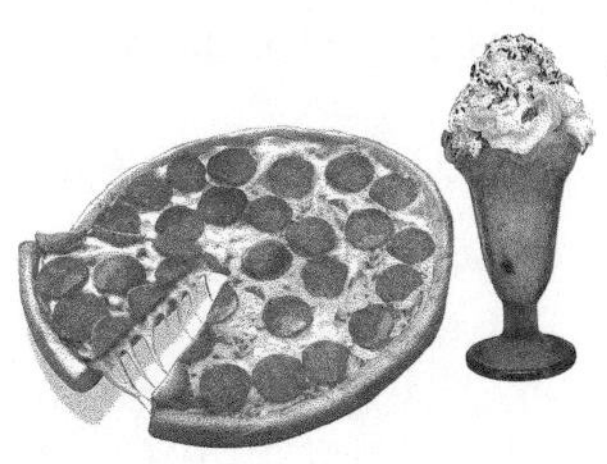

Chapter 2

My Life With Food

I am a middle-aged woman who has struggled with weight issues my entire life. I've tried every diet and swallowed every miracle pill. I had success; in fact I was so successful, I became obsessed. I have come full circle, but not without a lot of unnecessary suffering and pain.

I've tried every dieting aid from Dexatrim to *Body for Life*. I've devoured a dozen donuts at a time and have had a diet so pure it contained no refined sugar and a miniscule amount of fat. I almost failed ninth grade for continuously "bagging" gym because I literally hated exercise. But at 38, I taught seven aerobics classes and lifted weights 5 days a week in between taking power walks and playing golf. I've shoved an entire chocolate éclair in my mouth while no one was looking and I've stuck my fingers down my throat after inhaling one lousy wedge of pizza for dinner. The mirror that told me I looked great at 7 a.m. told me I looked fat at 7 p.m. At age 10 I thought people didn't like me because I was fat. At 40, I thought people didn't like me because I wasn't fat.

How It All Began

My first diet was at the age of 10. I tried an orange, egg and spinach diet. I made it up myself and, surprisingly, it was a pretty healthy combination – protein, fibrous carbs and a little fat. But boredom and lack of motivation took over and I found myself with a can of potato chips and a side of onion dip by the end of the second day.

Although I was never obese, every day I dreamed of being thin. I outgrew the Junior department at age 11 and being fat defined who I was and I didn't like myself. My worst clothing memory was not about zipping up a pair of pants or buying clothes in the plus size, but the trauma of not being able to wear boots. In the late '60's and early '70's high-heeled boots with zippered sides were popular. I was so excited when I was allowed to buy my first pair. Unfortunately, I couldn't zip them up. I bought them anyway and spent an hour trying to stretch the leather. I finally got them zipped and went to school, my calves numb from lack of circulation, only to be humiliated when the zipper ripped and I had to walk around school with my boot flapping.

The World's Worst Athlete

I felt abnormal and my self-esteem suffered (which was pretty darn low to start with). I had no self-confidence and was, or I felt I was, inept at everything I did. My body simply *hated* exercise, I thought. I didn't play sports and I nearly failed gym in high school because I would "cut" class. Gym was humiliating for me. I still can't forget the day my fellow students gave me a trophy at the end of ninth grade for the "School's Worst Athlete." I laughed as I always did in front of everyone, but I cried when I got home.

I was the second fattest girl in the Catholic school I attended. In those days being overweight was not as common as it is today. Of course, the fattest girl was my best friend. I used to love going to her house because her mom was *really* fat and they would always go eat at fast food restaurants (fast food was a rare treat in those days). Several years ago, my mom sent me a diary I had as a child. As I read it, I was amazed. While most preteen diaries are about boys my diary was all about food!

Today, we went to GINO's and I had a GINO GIANT!! It was so good.

❦

Today it snowed and we didn't have school. Yeah!! We went sledding and when we came home we had hot chocolate and toast with butter. I love dipping the toast in the hot chocolate. It tastes so good!!

My Life With Food

❦

Today, Daddy had to check on the store after church. I love going to the store when it's closed because I can play with the toys and raid the candy counter. My favorite ones are the chocolate turtles. I can have as much as I want!

I loved food and could eat a lot of it. My mom had a candy drawer (she still does, 30 years later – the same drawer!). I was the youngest of six kids with four brothers. Food was abundant, but it didn't last long. I remember hoarding candy and cookies on grocery day. I would hide chocolate bars in my dresser drawers and eat them alone in my room. I was worried that if I didn't hide them there wouldn't be any left. To this day, when I go to my mom's house, I still hit the candy drawer. *Honestly.* I can have the same candy in my house and I don't even look at it, but when I'm at Mom's the memories surface and I can't help myself.

As a child, I was always uncomfortable at the dinner table, just waiting for someone to comment on my eating. I learned to restrain myself at the table and then gorge food in solitude.

On the Boardwalk

One distinct food memory is eating food while walking on the Ocean City, Maryland, boardwalk. My parents and I would spend a few days at the beach. I was the youngest and my brothers and sister had left home, either married or at school. My parents would give me money to go on the boardwalk. I would be alone. No one was there to watch what I ate. Instead of going on rides or playing games, I would spend most of my time going from one food stand to another: cotton candy, french fries, caramel apples, fudge and snow cones. I would even go to breakfast by myself. I'd order pigs-in-a-blanket and sit at the counter, just my "friend" and me. I had friends when I was young, but my favorite friend was food.

I remember going to my sister-in-law's beach house in Wildwood, New Jersey, and buying a pound of fudge. I hid it under the bed, sneaked a piece from time to time, and by the end of the day it was gone.

By the next year's visit, I was reaching puberty and becoming aware of and upset about my extra weight. Being young and naive, I bought a box of Ayds with my allowance money (can you imagine calling a diet product "Ayds" today?). It was a diet chocolate that was supposed to suppress your appetite, popular in the late '60's, early '70's.

I also "borrowed" my older sister's two-piece bathing suit. I loved this suit. It had a big ruffled top and boy-cut, black and white polka-dot bottoms. Think of Gidget on her surfboard. My sister looked so groovy in it with her blonde pigtails and attractive curvy figure. You could just see her doing the "swim" or the "pony" at a beach bonfire party. My sister was my idol and I wanted to be just like her.

Well, I looked absolutely ridiculous. There I was, a chubby 12-year-old stuffed into my sister's fabulous suit. My big belly cutting across my nonexistent waistline, stretch marks between my flabby legs, and pigtails. I pranced around the beach feeling like Annette Funicello until one of my older brother's friends caught site of me and started laughing his head off. My bubble burst, reality set in and I went back to the beach house and ate the entire box of Ayds (you were only supposed to have two pieces at each meal), hiding them under the bed as I did the fudge. By the end of the first day, the box was empty and I was back on the boardwalk scoping out fudge and caramel apples. That was my first experience buying – and subsequently failing – a diet product.

The Pain of Rejection

Through adolescence I was always the last one to be picked for the team and rarely invited to "the parties." I envied everyone who was thinner than me. My brothers liked to tease me about my weight and my lack of athletic abilities. "Lard ass" was a nickname I painfully remember.

I was the type of kid who giggled uncontrollably when asked to do something that required agility or strength. We had a boat when I was young and I remember my brother and I were playing in the water and he wanted to put me on his shoulders and throw me off into the water like a diving board. Well, I couldn't get on his shoulders. He said, "Come on, get your fat ass out of the water!" I giggled and said, "I can't!" He dropped me, gave me a disgusted look and swam away. He stopped playing with me and it really hurt. I looked up to my brother and I disappointed him.

Not a very dramatic story, but I remember it vividly so it had an impact on me and experiences such as these defined who I was – or thought I was. I felt as though I couldn't do anything right. I associated all of the negative things I hated about myself, and why people didn't like me, with the fact that I wasn't thin. It was like an excuse for why I was the way I was. I thought I couldn't change myself, because I couldn't change my weight.

Feeling Unloved

Even though I had my share of teasing as a child, I really wasn't as fat as I remembered. I was more chubby than obese. But when you are a kid, it doesn't matter if you're 10 pounds overweight or 100, people don't accept you – or at least you feel like they don't accept you. You feel unloved and different and you wish you were anyone else but you.

My love of food dominated my childhood. I think as a child I wasn't overly obese because I got plenty of exercise even though I was not athletic. In those days, you weren't allowed to watch TV (not that there was anything good on anyway). You went outside and you came in for lunch and to go the bathroom. I can remember taking daylong bike rides or hiking through the woods behind our house. But even though I did the hiking and the biking, I was always the one who had to walk her bike up the hill, the last one to finish the race or fake an ankle sprain to cover up my inabilities.

As a child, I didn't feel loved and I always felt like a disappointment to everyone. Not that I wasn't loved; it's just that I never felt like I accomplished or I deserved anything. I was a people pleaser. I just wanted everyone to like me. I would do anything just to get people to like me. I'd give them money, allow myself to be used or be the brunt of their jokes. I'm not sure why I was like this. Looking back, I guess I always blamed myself for everything. If a neighborhood kid teased me or hurt me, I would run home to tell Mom. She would always tell me to just let it go and go back and play. You feel like everything is your fault. What did I do that made that person do that to me? After time you believe you aren't worth defending. I don't blame my mom though. She just wanted peace. So she taught her daughter to be the peacemaker too.

A Lifelong Preoccupation

Anyway, I've been obsessed with food all of my life. And by obsessed, I mean I didn't listen to the fullness in my stomach. I was preoccupied with food. I'd eat and eat and eat and sometimes I didn't know why I was eating so much, I just couldn't seem to help myself. It goes beyond "because it tastes so good." I've eaten half a cake while saying, "Yuck, I think the whipped-cream icing on this cake is bad." After a good food binge, I'd feel awful. Not only was I sick from the gluttony, I felt like a bad person. I always feared I wouldn't have enough food. Food called me even when I was full. I was not a selfish person, except when it came to food.

The Wild '70's

As a teenager, I discovered drugs. I was a child of the '70's and speed (diet pills) was available, almost acceptable. I remember going to an old senile doctor who would give out diet pills to just about anyone. I was cautious. I would only take them a few times a week to curb the excess amount of calories I would eat. I went overboard at age 19 right before my wedding to my first husband. I started taking a lot of diet pills during the six months of planning. I'm not sure if the primary reason was to look great going down the aisle or to mask the fact that deep down inside I had no clue what I was doing or why I was doing it.

I know at the time, my self-esteem was so low I was afraid no one else would love me. I was a trim 135 pounds but it didn't last long. Six months after I was married I shot up to 160 pounds even though I was still taking speed.

By that time I was into amphetamines. Methamphetamine, or "crank," as we called it then, was the most readily available. During this time I drank a lot and I was proud of it. Since I had the ability to consume large quantities of food without getting sick, I could also drink anyone under the table. I pretty much spent the late '70's drinking, drugging, smoking and eating. My addictive personality had the better of me and my future looked pretty bleak.

How I Tipped the Scales

A few years later I was pregnant with my first child. I remember when I was 21 and pregnant, I would stop at McDonald's on my way home from work and eat a Big Mac, fries and a chocolate shake. Then I'd go home and cook (and eat) dinner. What's important is not the fact that I ate so much, but *why* I ate so much and why I tried to hide it.

Fast food joints are an irresistible lure for a misguided lover of food. By yourself riding down the road, often without premeditation, we whip into the drive-thru and a few minutes later we're in the parking lot enjoying that almost orgasmic fix.

Afterwards, we feel guilty and ashamed. Almost like leaving the hotel room of an illicit lover. The most important thing is we not let anyone else know we did it. I can remember making sure I parked my car in the back of the parking lot in case someone I knew drove by – mimicking my habit of eating little at the dinner table and gorging on candy bars in my room. The action often gets worse as an adult when we have greater control of what we are "allowed" to consume. We have money, independence and access.

I stopped taking drugs (I wasn't a *total* idiot) and landed in the delivery room at a whopping 210 pounds. I remember the first thing I asked for when I woke up after a difficult delivery was a scale. Immediate postpartum depression set in when I still weighed 192 pounds! Of course, I lost some of the weight as the weeks went on, but I was older and wiser and now I had a child to care for. I didn't go back to drugs as a weight modifier. I had to find a diet that worked. But how can a diet work when you love food almost as much as life itself?

Life Changes

A year or so after my son was born, my marriage started to fall apart. Nothing was really different in our marriage, but I wanted to stop partying and grow up and my husband didn't. It's as if I woke up one day and realized I had this beautiful child and wanted the best for him. Even though I didn't deserve it, he did. I had little self-esteem and I knew I needed inner strength to get through a divorce. Being overweight was not going to help.

So I started jogging. I didn't really like it, but it was a time I could be by myself and clear my head. I developed a sense of strength and confidence I needed in order to get through the trauma of splitting up from my husband. It was during my run that I would map out my escape plan, review my past and relieve the fears that lay before me.

My parents were strict Catholics and weren't supportive of my decision. I was alone, just my son and me. I don't remember dieting during this time because I was always sick to my stomach, riddled with guilt and scared for the future. Still, I felt renewed and excited at the new life ahead of me.

From the Frying Pan to the Fire

As soon as the divorce papers were signed, I found myself, once again, in a bad relationship – this one worse than the first. After six abusive months, I finally had the courage to get rid of him. During my new trauma, food took a backseat to survival again.

I believe if I accepted the unhealthy and abusive relationships, food would have become my escape, my salvation. I think many women turn to food for comfort when they feel unable to control their lives or turn against food as a defense mechanism in an effort to control an uncontrollable situation.

Again, I freed myself from becoming a victim. I began a trend where I associated strength with weight. Keeping weight off and exercising became a coping technique for the trauma in my life. It was a survival tool.

As Long as I Was Thin

I kept running but with my heavy legs I could only plod along at what I thought was an embarrassing 11-minute mile. I started lifting weights, a concept not familiar to most females during the '80's. Weight lifting was a great motivator for me. Since I wasn't athletic, lifting weights gave me strength, both inner and outer, which I needed during that time. I was a novice and there wasn't a lot of support and education on the proper way to lift like there is now. I was a lonely, single, scared mother. I spent most of my time working and taking care of my son. The gym was my salvation.

There was a dark side to my life at that time. Although I wasn't doing drugs, I did experiment with bulimia out of fear of gaining weight. I tried to purge but, luckily, was unable to make myself throw up. I used to practice sticking my fingers down my throat, even asking a friend to help me do it. I even tried ipecac without success. I tried laxatives, but couldn't handle the untimely eruptions (I don't know how anyone can do that).

My Life With Food

I was always afraid of gaining weight. The scale became the only barometer to measure my self-worth. My weight seemed to be the only thing I could control. As long as I wasn't fat, I would be okay.

Off the Deep End

I remember a specific occasion when I was feeling guilty about my divorce, ashamed about my naivete with a psycho and weak from the stresses of life, I went on my lunch break and returned with six large chocolate éclairs from the local bakery. Alone, I ate every one of them in the parking lot. Then I returned to work, went to the bathroom and gagged unsuccessfully.

This process became a habit. I was terrified of my future. I didn't like being alone and I still didn't like myself. I would resist my desire to overeat but then temporarily relieve myself with a food binge only to hate myself for being weak.

Emotional binging is a trancelike experience. The world around you becomes still and the eating process is methodical. It's as if you are in a dream and then you come back to reality. When you wake up, you realize what you have done and go, "Ugh! What the hell have I done!" My self-esteem was very low and I became vulnerable and desperate. Trying to find love. Trying to avoid being alone.

Respectfully Yours

I started to get recognition at my job and it made me feel a little better about myself. It was the first time I felt anyone gave me respect. I got promoted and I actually thought I might be good at something. I started to get my act together and made some changes in my life. I stopped trying to find love in all the wrong places and focused on the positive aspects of my life. I stopped going to bars and focused on being a better mom. I started to care more about myself. I actually started to believe I could be worthy of someone's love and was willing to be content with myself until I found it – if I found it.

My White Knight

Then I met my husband, a good guy. It seems you only find

love when you aren't looking for it. But I think it's that good guys find self-respect appealing and for the first time I didn't appear desperate for love. I was so happy I was able to let my guard down. While I was still carrying a lot of emotional baggage, I was happy – at least for a while.

My husband and I had the same love for food. I stopped exercising and started eating. Oh did we eat well together! I remember the first year of marriage we would cook together and go out to eat often. Our leisure activities were always about food. I remember one Sunday we spent the entire day making homemade donuts. I think we made five dozen and ate copious amounts of them until we couldn't shove another one in.

I gained 15 pounds and then I started having babies again – always a good excuse to ignore your weight. After the birth of my third and last child, I was 33 years old and I looked at myself in the mirror. I didn't like what I saw. I felt fat, old and saggy. I wasn't really that overweight, but the perception of myself was very bad.

Love Is Truly Blind

Even though my husband would love me no matter how heavy I got, I didn't believe he could. I had done a good job of covering it up but my self-esteem was still bad and it was hurting our marriage. It drove my husband crazy when I put myself down or turned myself inside out trying to please him – instead of asking for what I wanted. Everyone else in my life took advantage of my need to please. But my husband detested it. I needed a self-esteem overhaul and the only way I knew how to do it was to lose weight.

The problem was finding the time. I was working full time; had three children, one in diapers and one in Little League; and a house to take care of.

I started running again. I worked up to running three miles at a nearby park after work. I knew if I came home I would never get the chance. My husband was very supportive and started to motivate himself as well. I tried to eat healthy foods and I was on working mom overload. I would fall asleep as soon as the kids got to bed – so I stopped eating at night. The weight came off, but the obsession didn't stop.

As the kids got older and my life settled down, I continued to exercise and weight train. Exercise and weight training became an obsession because it kept me from feeling depressed. If I didn't work out daily, I would end up feeling worthless by the end of the day.

My Obsession Grows

The older I got, the more obsessed I became about how I looked. Food continued to be a problem. I forced myself on a daily basis to stick to a limited diet. I had to keep a journal every day. I would count every fat, carbohydrate and protein gram and note my weight, body fat and exercise/weight training routine. I would weigh myself numerous times a day. I was obsessed with it. I would freak out if I gained a pound or two. If I gave myself a day off, I would be totally out of control.

Going to Sunday dinner at Grandma's was my free eating pass. I allowed myself to eat and I ate into oblivion. Her food was delicious and ample, and eating was encouraged. I'd eat and eat and then get totally depressed on the 45-minute drive home with my pants unbuttoned, beating myself up for being so gluttonous.

I lived in fear of food. The negative memories of my love for food as a child and the damage it did to my self-esteem haunted me. Even though I conquered my weight problem, I was afraid of going out of control unless I forced myself not to overeat on a daily basis. I was afraid to let my guard down. I was still obsessed with food, dieting and my body. I thought I was successful only because I was extremely disciplined. Undisciplined, I would become the chubby kid I didn't like again.

Who Am I?

People around me thought I was just a healthy person. Some were inspired or envious or admired my dedication. For eight years I ate healthy and exercised, but every day was a struggle. The struggle became easier with time, but I was always depriving myself and exercising to the point of exhaustion to "work off" the cheating I had done. I felt like a pig when I overate or ate any unhealthy foods. I might as well have weighed 250 pounds.

I would hate myself because I gave in to my weakness, then I'd feel sorry for myself because I couldn't eat like everyone else. I would feel sorry for myself because I couldn't look like the women in the magazines whose diet and exercise programs weren't as strict as mine. I would document my stringent food allowance and excessive exercise routines, but beat myself up because I had cheated and had a piece of pizza one night. "Aha, you weak person. No wonder you don't look like them!"

There were times when I felt pretty good about myself and times I felt like an ugly, fat, bad person. My attitude revolved around how much and what I ate and how often I exercised. While people were jealous of me, I was jealous of the people who were happy with themselves even though they wore a size 14. Sure they admitted they could lose 10 pounds, but they were happy with themselves and they had more important things to worry about.

Obsession Limits Your Life

I became so consumed with my quest for the perfect body that, to a certain extent, I stopped living. I was totally self-absorbed in the quest.

The first four hours of my day revolved around obsessing. I had to start the day off with a rigorous exercise program. But, I had to plan that around when and what I ate.

If I was doing aerobics, I had to eat and then wait two hours before exercising. If I was lifting, I had to eat a little for energy; wait; then lift; then eat a post-workout meal that contained a certain proportion of protein and carbohydrates. I used to eat only at home, where I could maintain my rigid diet.

I worshipped my eating time. I couldn't just eat something at the mall. And I had to eat on a time schedule. I had to stop what I was doing, go home and have my "power" food. I spent about $100 a month on supplements. I would read about every new supplement and try every new miracle weight loss theory in search of perfection.

Obsession Becomes Career

The obsession turned into a career. Since I had to eat, sleep and exercise my quest, I quit a lucrative professional career to become an aerobics instructor and personal trainer. Changing careers where my body became an advertisement for my business really put the pressure on me. I always felt like I was being judged by my appearance. People around me started to go out of their way to excuse themselves for the piece of cake they were eating or put themselves down because they hadn't worked out in a while. I started to feel very uncomfortable. I felt like an outsider, like my body defined who I was and any flaws I showed would be flaws in me. So much of who I was became my body.

I had already met a realistic potential, but when I tried and tried and couldn't meet my unrealistic potential I started to backslide. I had nowhere to go but down.

My Obsession Spreads

I loved teaching aerobics and I wanted to inspire others. Even though I was in denial over my obsession, I wanted to share the positive side of my behavior. I wanted to introduce people to the great feeling of regular exercise. I also had empathy for those who struggled unsuccessfully to lose weight. Unlike a lot of professional trainers, I knew their pain and I knew it was hard to change and even harder to *believe* you could change. I could relate to their pain and I thought I could give them hope by helping them to change.

I really enjoyed my career for a while, but then I started to blame myself for not inspiring others enough to get them to reach their goals. Because of society's pressures to be "thin" and the promises made in diet books, aids and magazine articles (lose 10,15, 20 pounds in 30 days on our "all you can eat" diet) I didn't succeed at getting them to meet their unrealistic goals.

Now, not only was I beating myself up for not meeting my own goals, I now felt responsible for others not meeting their goals. I felt like I was capitalizing on people's weaknesses and emotions. I quit the personal training business. I felt like a failure in just one more aspect of life.

The Moment of Truth

Even though I was visibly successful for years, I hadn't overcome my problem. Drugs, life trauma and an unhealthy obsession had kept me from being fat. But throughout my life, the driving force was my psychological need to not be fat. It was a survival tool. There were periods in my life when I needed to be strong and the only way I could be strong was to be thin.

I fought the food demon for 30 years. Not many days went by when I didn't think about the repercussions of what I was eating. Some days I was able to control the demon. On others it reared its ugly head. As the obsession grew my self-worth deteriorated until it nearly destroyed me. The unrealistic demands I placed on myself took control and sabotaged every positive thing I did. I hit rock bottom and knew I had to stop the madness.

Figuring It Out

Sorting out the childhood psychological garbage helped, but it wasn't the answer. I was looking for answers in all the wrong places and the quest had consumed me.

I knew I had to stop using the mirror as a gauge for acceptance of myself. I had to make food my friend again. It was very hard to do. I was so afraid of going back to the chubby kid that I hated. Even though my weight loss triumphs did little to improve my self-esteem, at least I wasn't fat. I was able to control my weight, but at what price?

I had to stop expecting so much from my body. After all, I turned 40 and I couldn't control aging. Future expectations were only going to be more difficult to meet. I was never going to have the body of a 25-year-old. I had to put it all behind me.

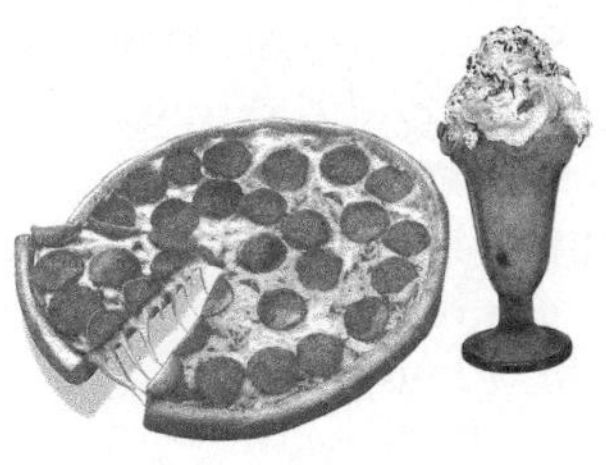

Chapter 3

How I Set Myself Free – and How You Can Too!

Once I recognized and learned to control my obsessive behaviors, I found the answer. After 30 years of fighting my demons, I have won.

I wanted to stop the obsession to have a perfect body without transforming back into the chubby kid. In all the years that I worked out and ate healthy, the primary reason was not for my health or that it was something I liked to do. I did it to lose weight, fight depression or try to improve my self-esteem. I was dieting, exercising and obsessing in a very destructive way. I wanted to eat healthy because I chose to, not because I had to. I wanted to exercise, not because I had to, but because it *felt good*. I needed to moderate how much I ate because I didn't like being overly full.

So How Did I Do It?

What I decided was to strive to be the type of person that I was *really* jealous of. The ones I always thought were different from me – a person who eats what they want and stops eating when they are full. The ones who get regular exercise as an enjoyable part of their life, not because they *have* to do it. A person that is content with an imperfect body.

Most importantly I wanted to set myself free from my destructive, obsessive behaviors. The negative way I thought about myself, the negative way I behaved and the negative way I lived my life.

I spent my life dieting and obsessing with impossible expectations because I thought I could never be one of *them*. I decided to change my direction and follow a different path. I decided I would start believing and living like I *was* one of them. So I taught myself how and set myself free.

How About You?

Are you obsessing? Do you believe that you have a food problem you can't control, or that exercise is something you could never want to do? Does the mirror validate your worth? Are you constantly trying new diet theories, products and pills and then beating yourself up because they fail to meet your expectations? Do you blame yourself? You can keep trying, but one thing is for sure. You will never solve your problem unless you get over your obsession. You must believe you can become someone who doesn't have an issue with their weight or their body and who lives a healthy lifestyle because it's what they *want* to do.

So how did I do it? How can you do it? Saying it and doing it are very different things. It doesn't come miraculously but it's a lot easier than any diet or crazy exercise contraption or pill.

And it's liberating. After all, someone will always appear to be better looking than you but you are the only one that really cares. You can solve your weight problem by ridding yourself of your negative behaviors and finding acceptance with food and your body. You can learn to eat right and exercise not because you *have* to do it, but because you *want* to do it. And that's what I am going to teach you.

9 Steps to The NEW You

I've formulated a nine-step program that follows my journey of failure, success and, most importantly, my liberation from my weight problems. I share my extensive emotional, mental and physical expertise I learned from my research as well as the practical school of hard knocks. I try to point out the reasons we are overweight to help you identify the reasons you have weight issues. I believe I've come up with a program that can truly change how you view yourself and your life – ***forever***.

How I Set Myself Free – and How You Can Too!

The 9 Steps isn't just another way to lose weight. The program transforms you. The result is a NEW You.

There are no gimmicks. There isn't a formula. You don't have to be a purist to make it work. But you do need to get educated and openly explore the reasons you have weight issues in order to figure out what you can do about it.

Diets Don't Work

Before we even begin the 9 Steps to The New You, we need to eliminate the confusion and misrepresentation of ridiculous promises, guarantees, theories and miracles developed by the diet industry. I'll explain why diets work or don't work and why exercise gadgets and miracle pills don't work either, regardless of the "proven" results claimed in books and on television. If you can believe diets, gadgets and pills aren't the answer, hopefully, you'll stop buying, trying and failing.

Solving Your Weight Issues and Wanting a Healthy Lifestyle – *Forever*

How can you become a person without weight issues? You need to identify your problem, find a solution to your problem and then implement that solution. We've heard enough about what we should be doing and we aren't doing it. You need to be mentally ready for change in order to physically change it. You need to understand your feelings, identify the behaviors resulting from those feelings and, most importantly, you need to believe you can change and you must *want* to change. *Then* you can move forward and start the journey to success.

Once you have established where you went wrong and why, the 9 Steps will help you figure out the solution. It will help you learn to:

- Overcome negative thinking and unrealistic expectations with regards to your weight, your body and yourself.
- Have a healthy relationship with food by not letting food control you and learn how to make food your friend again.
- Live a healthy lifestyle because it's what you *want* to do not because you feel you *have* to do it.
- Implement the actual physical behaviors required to live a healthier lifestyle. With your new attitude you will succeed because you want it and are empowered to do it.

The program prepares you for change and then shows you how to change for realistic, obtainable results – results that go way beyond a number on a scale.

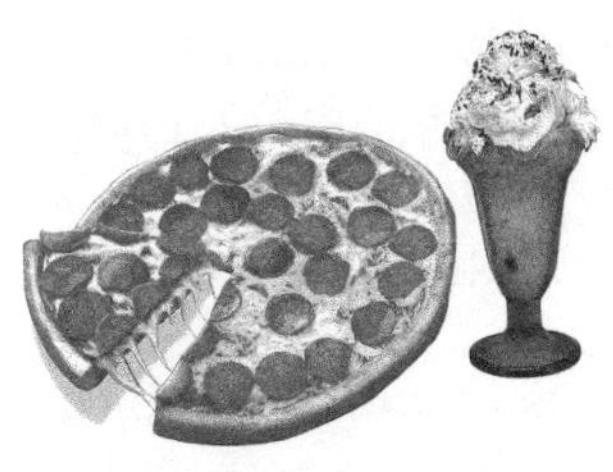

Chapter 4

Revealing the Truths Behind Diets, Gadgets and Gurus

Have you tried all the diets, gadgets and pills claiming easy, guaranteed weight loss but have experienced little or no results? Have you listened and applied all the so-called "expert" theories and still haven't met your goals? Have you gotten depressed and blamed yourself? I have. Maybe it's time we realize the problem isn't us. It's the diets, gadgets and pills.

Popular diets and products don't work without the fundamental elements of caloric intake, willpower and self-discipline. The same obstacles we have been dealing with for years only now they have made the process even more difficult by confusing us with ridiculous "scientific" theories and gibberish. And in our desperation for a solution we are gullible enough to believe it. We get hopeful and then when we fail, we blame ourselves. Or, we go into denial and blame something else.

The only solution we know works is to eat fewer calories, exercise more, or both. It's the proven method that works and it's actually the easiest way.

But people say, "I've tried that and it doesn't work." "I need something to follow that doesn't require me to count calories or have willpower." "I can't seem to find the time to exercise." It's hard to accept but the more educated you are, the more likely you will be able to let go of the notion that there is some "magic" way to help you lose weight.

The Ultimate Truth

There is no way around it. You have to reduce caloric intake or increase caloric expenditure through exercise. That requires some motivation and willpower. Fad diets and products only camouflage the reality.

There are thousands of gadgets, pills and books that promise to give you the body of your dreams with little effort and without dieting. There are contraptions that burn mega calories without effort; pills that work while you sleep; and foods that give you unlimited energy. We want to believe what we are being told because it all sounds so magical, even logical. We don't want to lose weight the old-fashioned – only proven – way, so we look to miracles or theories that don't really exist.

It's all about the gimmick. What gimmick will sell a book on how to lose weight without effort. It's about the gadget. What gadget will guarantee you to lose 30 pounds in 30 days or your money back. It's about the magic pill that melts away fat while you sleep. It's a theory that explains it's not how much you eat, but what you eat that's your problem.

It's about someone making a truckload of money from suckers like us because they know we will try anything and buy everything in an effort to lose weight.

You're Not Alone

Don't get me wrong. You aren't the only one. When I say "we," I don't mean "you." I mean "me" and probably some of you. Marketing techniques can be so convincing that I still find myself searching for the "magic" even though I know better. I believe because I want to believe. Just the other day I stayed up for the late news so I could listen to the review of a "scientific breakthrough" – *pantyhose that reduce cellulite!* A growing trend is to bolster news ratings by advertising new diet products that aren't worthy of being buried in the back of the *National Enquirer.*

I've bought and read all the best sellers that claim they have found the magic eating plan that guarantees you'll lose all the weight you want and still eat your favorite foods. These books sell by tearing apart the food pyramid using scientific sleight of hand to justify ridiculous theories. Some include extreme eating changes.

I used to be one who found counting calories too difficult, yet I'd readily eliminate entire categories of food from my diet. Now really, which is "easier" – paying attention to the amount of calories you eat or forever giving up carbohydrates from your diet?

Most of the new diet theories are nothing more than complex gibberish. You don't need a 300-page book to tell you that you can lose weight by not eating sugar.

One Lie After Another

I saw the cover of a magazine that said, *"Sexy Thighs By Summer Guaranteed!"* The article profiled a beautiful 20-something fitness instructor with legs to die for and not a speck of cellulite to be seen. Hanging on to that last hope, I buy the magazine and anxiously turn to the article that will reveal the magic secret to thinner thighs. Disappointed, what I find are three exercises – a squat, a lunge and a donkey kick, using 3-pound dumbbells. Hey, wait a minute! These are the same routines I have been doing for seven years only with an 85-pound barbell on my back! When will I ever learn!

So was the article wrong to suggest these exercises can improve your thighs? No, of course not. What's wrong is they foster unrealistic expectations of results. The gorgeous model with the great legs lures us into believing our legs can look like hers too!

But realistically, if they showed a 175-pound woman whose thighs were reduced one-eighth inch in eight weeks, no one would be lured into buying the magazine. Our expectations, our desires, are to be someone we are not and do it in 30 days or less.

Lies Prey Upon Our Souls

With every diet, product or pill we try without success, our mental attitude about ourselves gets worse. Why can't I be like that person? Why am I such a failure? You look in the mirror and the image of yourself is worse than the day before. Our self-esteem takes yet another nosedive and we make ourselves feel better by curling up with a gallon of Rocky Road and a shovel.

Instead of blaming our weaknesses for not getting the advertised results, we should be blaming the marketing strategists who have been playing with our heads and making money at our expense.

It's Not All Bad

Of course, not all of the diet aids are bad. Some are helpful in reaching our goals. I've had experiences with them all. Maybe you have. And if you haven't, maybe my stories will convince you not to waste your money or time or drain your self-esteem.

So let's examine the most popular diet aids, put them in reasonable perspective, keep the good stuff and toss the rest out of our minds. Once we've accomplished this, then we can move forward to a different, better and easier way to tackle the problem.

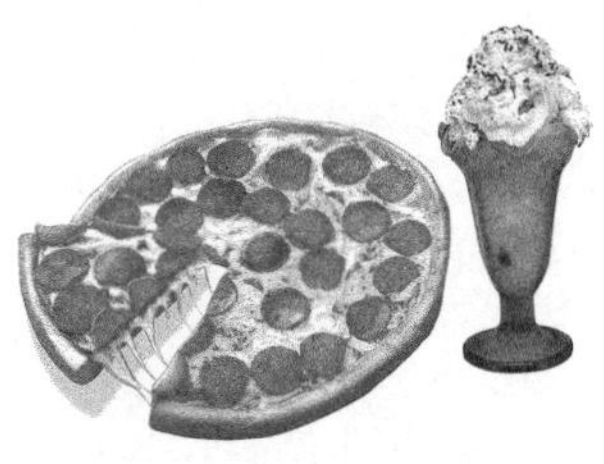

Chapter 5

Dissecting the Diets

A new era in dieting is evolving. After over 1200 books have been written on the subject of "the best diet to lose weight" nutritionists, doctors and psychologists are now coming to one united conclusion. *Diets don't work.* And by following them, our country is only getting fatter. Eighty percent of the diet books were published since 1997. We don't know what to eat any more. We just keep buying into the solution of the week and when we fail we try a new one. While some of the information is worthwhile, usually it is delivered in an extreme, sometimes dangerous package.

If you can learn more about how these diets really work, you might be able to put them behind you and get back to reality. Let's take a look at some of the more popular diets and see what's *really* going on with their theories.

Dieting by Process of Elimination

Before we begin, it's important to remind you that food (calories) only comes in four categories – protein, fat, carbohydrate and alcohol.

Low-Fat Diets

"It's the fat that makes you fat" was the motto of the low-fat diet revolution. Eat less fat and you will lose weight. Many of us did, for a while. We cut back on the chips, the fried foods, and the oils and we all started losing weight. Fat became a dirty word and carbohydrates became the good guy.

Low-fat diets work because, theoretically, if you reduce the fat in your diet, you reduce calories. Fat has the most calories per gram (nine versus four for carbohydrate and protein). If you reduce the fat in your diet, you will lose weight. The medical community provided an added incentive with the recommendation that a diet low in fat was beneficial to our health. A low-fat diet continues to be the most beneficial to our health, but somehow things went wrong.

The message got distorted and soon "It's the fat that makes you fat" turned into "Eat as much as you want as long as it isn't fat." We all started to gain weight again. You know why? *It's not the fat that makes you fat – it's the calories.*

Soon we were all carbohydrate binging. The food industry started taking the fat out of our snack foods and we gobbled them up guilt free. In most cases, the fat replacement was sugar. The end result was we weren't eating fat, but we were eating just as many, if not more, calories in sugar!

Somehow protein got a bad rap as well. Most fat in animal protein sources is saturated fat and contains cholesterol. Everyone was avoiding fat and protein. The only food option left was carbohydrates.

When we started gaining weight again, we started to remove more and more fat from our diet but we were still gaining weight.

High-Fat Diets

Coming to the rescue was Dr. Robert C. Atkins. He pronounced it's not the fat that's making us fat, it's the carbohydrates! Based on the declining success of the low-fat diets, he was partially right. The problem was, he threw the baby out with the bath water. Instead of advocating adding more fat and protein back into our diet, he said carbohydrates were the "bad guy." He preached that nearly eliminating carbohydrates and living mostly on fat and protein was the solution. So now everyone started having bacon for breakfast, a hunk of cheese for lunch and a T-bone for dinner.

Hooray, we thought, we can all eat fat again! The only catch was we couldn't eat the carbohydrates with it. Think about it; what's a cheese steak without the chewy Italian roll that goes with it; a great meat sauce without the pasta; cheese without crackers! Not to mention, no french fries to go with that Quarter Pounder with cheese (but don't forget to take off the roll!). And let's not forget that sugar is a carbohydrate. No chocolate, cake, cookies, ice cream, not even fruits or yogurts!

Alas, There Was No Magic

Everyone who stayed on the diet magically started to lose weight. We concluded, "You see, it *was* the carbohydrates that were making us fat!" But there was no magic. You lose weight following the diet because *you eat fewer calories.* The clincher to this diet is that you get so sick of eating just protein and fat that you lose your appetite. But if you are eating so much fat, how can you be eating fewer calories you ask? Well, if you consider what I previously said, what can you really eat and how long before you get sick of eating it!

Without adding carbohydrates to the fat, the only way you can eat fat is by itself or with protein. You can have a piece of meat or fish. You can add some cheese, mayonnaise, sour cream to it or you could just gnaw on a stick of butter if you wanted. I get sick just thinking about it.

Absent from this diet was fiber, fruits and many vegetables. Not only that, following his diet would increase the risk of cardiovascular disease and some cancers.

Dr. Atkins says you can eat as much of this stuff as you want and still lose weight. The problem is you can only eat so much of it before you stop wanting it. If you stay on the diet, it does work. It's easy to eat four pieces of bread (about 360 calories) with dinner, but try eating three chicken breasts (about 360 calories) instead. It's very hard to do without feeling sick.

Hopeful, But Disappointed

I tried the Atkins Diet. I was excited too! Maybe I couldn't lose those last 10 pounds because I wasn't eating enough fat! Could this be the answer I've been looking for? I followed the diet for one week. The first couple of days, I still wanted my ice cream and bread, but I felt energetic and I wasn't hungry. By the end of the week, however, I felt downright nauseated and I didn't want to eat any of the "allowable" foods. I was also fatigued. I didn't want fat; I didn't want protein; I just wanted a bowl of cereal!

The Pizza and Ice Cream Diet

Some people (mostly men) are successful at losing weight because they are meat lovers. It's like putting me on a diet where I could only eat sweets. Yeah, I could do that! This is the guy who claims he eats a pound of bacon every morning. While a pound of bacon sounds like a lot of calories, a pound of bacon is typically about 600-700 calories after cooking. That's really not an excessive amount of breakfast calories for a grown man. But, it is difficult to eat a pound of bacon without feeling sick. Besides, if he really is eating this way, I hope he is putting a down payment on his bypass surgery!

The diet isn't new. Dr. Atkins originally marketed his diet almost 30 years ago. My recollection is the diet was popular with wrestlers and boxers who needed to qualify for a weight class because high protein diets produce fast scale loss. The reason is that the lack of carbohydrates rids your body of water. As soon as you resume eating, the scale weight comes back.

The Gold Rush Begins

Along with Dr. Atkins came other books jumping on the low-carbohydrate bandwagon. *The Carbohydrate Addicts Diet, Sugar Busters, Protein Power* and others offered similar messages – ***carbohydrates are bad***. "We've become a nation addicted to carbohydrates," they claim, "and that's why we're all fat."

How ridiculous. If a food isn't a fat or a protein, it's a carbohydrate. So why don't we call it the food addict's diet? If you cut out carbohydrates, you're cutting out nearly every enjoyable food option – bread, potatoes, pasta, chocolate, cake, cookies, brownies, rice, etc. If you have a diet that restricts most carbohydrates, especially the yummy ones, you are bound to lose weight. Why? *Because you eat fewer calories!* But how boring. Not only that, fruit and most vegetables are restricted as well.

Oprah, the Fad Diet Guru

When I heard Oprah complain on national television that she couldn't have her apple because it was a carbohydrate, I wanted to jump through the television and strangle her! Come on, Oprah! You are respected by millions of people as a smart lady. How can you be that gullible! What's more, she didn't lose any weight!

It's not because she can't lose weight on low-carbohydrate diets – she can't *stay* on the diet. Is it because she is a carbohydrate addict? No, but like most of us she loves food. Since most foods are carbohydrates, she can't control her weight because she is eating more calories than she needs, not because she is eating more carbohydrates. Mentally, she probably wants carbohydrates even more because she is being told she can't have them!

Why Make It Even Harder?

High-protein, low-carbohydrate diets work. They work if you have the willpower to stay on them. But isn't it easier just to modify your diet so that you can eat all foods, but less of them? If you can't stop eating a half a bag of Doritos, then how are you going to eliminate every snack food as well as all other carbohydrates?

The Magic Combination Diets

Low-fat diets weren't working, high-fat diets weren't working, so along come the magic combination diets. These diets claim all food components are good – protein, fat and carbohydrate as long as we eat them in the right combination. A "magic formula" that, if followed, will allow you to eat all the foods you want and still lose weight. Sounds great! But alas again, there really wasn't any magic.

The Zone Diet

The Zone Diet, developed by Dr. Barry Sears, promised to deliver the *"most powerful means ever discovered to help people achieve that state of optimal good health, physical performance, and mental alertness." The Zone Diet* book has spent months on the best-seller list and he has written and marketed other *Zone* books. Hollywood has embraced his diet. *The Zone Diet* take-out food in Hollywood is the latest rage.

Dr. Sears says bad eicosanoids are the culprit behind our society's ills and obesity. Bad eicosanoids, he says, are caused by excessive carbohydrate intake and eating in "the zone" will give you good eicosanoids. Eicosanoids produce *"a powerful hormone that controls every vital physiological function in the human body."* Eicosanoids are controlled by dietary fat so if we aren't consuming enough dietary fat our eicosanoids aren't able to do their job.

He also claims that high-carbohydrate diets make you fat. Follow his easy plan, Sears claims, and you will lose weight permanently. Eat in "the zone" and you will *"overcome controllable ill health, weight problems and feel physically and mentally alert."*

He says the USDA food guidelines are "dead wrong" and sets out to prove it.

Have We Found the Holy Grail?

Sounds pretty shocking and impressive. Dr. Sears has discovered the problem with our diets and sets out to explain his theory for permanent weight loss and optimal health.

I bought and read this book and found that what he said and what he delivered were two different things. His comparisons to other diets are misleading and while it's true you will lose weight, the diet itself is nothing more than a low-calorie diet. No secrets. No magic.

The theory that carbohydrates make you fat is unfounded. His methods work because most of us are eating too many carbohydrate *calories*. Reduce carbohydrates and you eat fewer calories. If you eat fewer calories, you lose weight. If you lose weight, you will feel better and become healthier.

The Real Scoop

Let me explain. Yes, he says you can have all the foods as long as you eat in a 30 percent protein, 30 percent fat and 40 percent carbohydrate ratio. But the catch is how much you can eat revolves around the precise amount of protein requirements your body needs.

He makes the food percentage equation easy by using a "block" system. It sounds scientific, but the "blocks" are simply cleverly disguised calories. I'll give you a scenario to help explain how the diet really works.

According to Dr. Sears' calculation, my allowable protein number is 88 grams per day. Therefore I can eat 352 protein calories a day. These 352 calories are supposed to represent 30 percent of my total caloric intake for the day. Eighty-eight grams of protein is about three servings a day. Most healthy diets recommend a serving of protein at each meal. So there's nothing wrong or excessive about the protein number.

Add another 352 calories for my 30 percent fat calorie allowance. Thirty percent of fat calories is also recommended by USDA and other dietary guidelines. No big news there.

The "magic" comes from the allowable carbohydrate calories. You can have 40 percent of your calories from carbohydrates. Using 88 grams of protein (30 percent) as your starting point and another 30 percent allowed for fat, 40 percent of total daily calories equals 503 calories per day in allowable carbohydrates.

Let's add up the numbers using calories as the measurement instead of grams or percentages:

Protein	352 calories
Fat	352 calories
Carbohydrates	503 calories
Total	1207 calories

Therefore, on *The Zone Diet*, my total daily allowable calories is 1207. I about fell off my chair when I figured this out! Of course you are going to lose weight, you're on a low calorie diet!

The only real difference between *The Zone Diet* and the USDA Daily Recommended diet (which he denounces) is that you have to eat fewer servings of carbohydrates. In other words, eat less chips, soda and cookies. Isn't that essentially what the USDA recommends for weight loss?

Out of "The Zone"

But we already tried low-calorie diets and we said, "It's too hard!" So why would we be so excited about a diet that not only restricts the foods we love, but makes the process even more complicated and confusing?

Why? Because he hides the inevitable truth behind impressive sounding psychobabble.

The *Zone* theory is debunked by most nutrition specialists. Pat Kendall, Ph.D., R.D., concluded *"the metabolic pathways presented in "The Zone Diet" which supposedly connect diet, insulin, glucagon and eicosanoids may sound impressive, but simply do not exist in standard nutrition or biochemistry text. The idea that The Zone Diet, or any diet, completely controls the secretion of insulin and glucagon is not supported by the relationship between nutrition and endocrinology."*

Body for Life

Body for Life, by Bill Phillips, is another "magic combination" best-seller. His diet is similar to *The Zone* but he adds another "magic" component of precise exercise, eating frequency and weight training. Bill Phillips was my hero. I read his book. I have his video. I drank his shakes and I took his supplements. And I even waited every other month with anticipation for his next issue of *Muscle Media*. Within six months I hated him. (No I don't hate anyone, just the things they do.) Bear with me while I vent. My *Body for Life* experience brought me to the brink of my obsession.

On the Right Track

Bill Phillips was on the right track. He advocates good nutrition, regular exercise and weight training. All great recommendations, but his business sense turned his motives into a lucrative money-making marketing campaign including the sales of his body-building supplements.

The problem with *Body for Life* is he turns his healthy living philosophy into a precise formula with expectations of unrealistic, nearly impossible, results.

The Challenge

In addition to his best-selling book, *The Body for Life* "Challenge" is one of his marketing strategies. He offers $100,000 to the person who achieves the best results in three months using his methods. The results are quite stunning. But are the results really possible?

First of all, Phillips is practically perfect. He's good-looking and has an awesome body. Plus he's smart, disciplined and a terrific businessman. That is problem number one. He's intimidating.

He asks you to have a "future vision." Then he has you write down a goal. A suggested goal would be, "I want to lose 20 pounds of fat and gain 10 pounds of muscle in 12 weeks." That's *some* goal. Okay, so the goal he wants you to meet is a bit aggressive. Phillips is a driven man. In his view, tough goals mean better results.

The Trouble in River City

Now here is the disturbing part. He wants you to make that goal a "promise." *"If you break your promise, you are breaking your word. This promise must be treated as earnestly as a vow you make to your spouse. Or to your child."* Wow, talk about putting pressure on oneself! I understand his intent is to get you to seriously focus on the transformation. If you are successful, he says.

"You will unleash enormous energy and potential. That potential emptiness created by self-deception will become filled with strength, certainty, and, yes, confidence, if you honor self-promises."

The result is wonderful if you succeed. But what if you don't? How do you feel about yourself then? Are you then deceitful, weak, dishonorable? Suicidal perhaps?

The Quest for My "Body for Life"

It all started when we got a complimentary issue of Bill Phillips' magazine, *Muscle Media,* in the mail. The transformation pictures were stunning. I was in pretty good shape, but I was in my obsessive phase and still hated my body. I especially loathed my cellulite. I worked for years to get rid of my excess weight and cellulite but it seemed that no matter what I did, I couldn't get better results.

Was this the best I could be? I was frustrated and desperate. With Bill Phillips' powerful inspirational message and unique plan, maybe I could be transformed into someone I thought I couldn't be! Maybe with Bill Phillips' help I could achieve what I thought was the impossible. He showed me proof that he could turn a Pillsbury Doughboy into Hercules in only three months!

There was a woman in the Transformation Challenge whose "before" body looked sort of like mine (if I had bad hair, a sad face, an excruciatingly tight bathing suit, sagging posture and pasty skin). Her after picture was awesome. That's what I wanted! Bill Phillips assured me I could look like her if I followed his program. What's more, he said the diet would get rid of my cellulite! I had to go for it. It's now or never. I was ready for the challenge!

My husband was even on board. We ordered his *Body for Life* video; we bought his book and his supplements and began our journey.

I Tried, I **Really** *Tried*

I followed his program as closely as I could. I had a modest goal of losing only 5 pounds and two percent body fat. I followed his recommended plan. I had my journal, I gave myself daily affirmation and I ate six times a day. I drank one or two of his Myoplex Lite protein shakes every day. I calculated the time I ate, the time I exercised, and how much I slept. I followed his weight-lifting schedule and critiqued my technique constantly.

I wasn't perfect, but he said in his book that even the people who win the transformation admit to cheating once in a while. I kept up the program as best I could but it was very difficult to stick to his demanding regimen. The weight training and aerobics weren't so bad, but the food schedule was a page from hell. I had to eat every couple of hours each day and it had to be something very nutritious. I felt like a breast-feeding baby! What's more, every time I stopped to eat I wanted to eat more than my allowance, even though I wasn't even hungry when I had to eat!

Since I couldn't be in the kitchen all day preparing my next nutritious meal, I sometimes relied on his nutrition bars. These awful tasting bars came in second only to the pasty, tasteless protein shakes that are marketed as "delicious." The only thing good about his shakes is that after ingesting one I wasn't hungry because I was sick.

My husband was on the diet with me. He would often be stuck in meetings that would last hours or a full day. What was he supposed to do look at his watch and say, "Sorry folks, I've got to go get my protein shake. It's feeding time!"

Not Making Sense

Not being able to exercise more than I wanted was also difficult. He says we should do aerobic exercise for 20 minutes at high intensity three times a week– "no more, no less;" weight training was to take no more than 46 minutes. Anything else would compromise the transformation results.

But what if your current lifestyle is physically intensive? What about people who are avid joggers, who walk a golf course, play tennis or racquetball? What about people who enjoy hiking, long distance biking and other activities? Do they have to cut back on their activities during the "transformation"?

It's like his way is the *only* way. There are no options. Assuming you are allowed to exercise for more than 20 minutes, can you then eat more? Can you eat more and still be "transforming"? Can I still transform if it takes me 58 minutes instead of 46 minutes to weight lift? Common sense says yes, but he never talks about it. One is left to believe exercising any more is counterproductive. Does this make sense?

One day a week you are allowed to take a day off. Eat anything and everything you want. You suffer for six days, and on the seventh day you eat; and eat, and eat, and eat. At least I did. Say "go," and I "go." Looking back on my 12 weeks of endless suffering, I most likely re-ate the calories I saved being good all week on my free day. I guess maybe that's why I failed. Regardless, fasting and binging is not my idea of building a healthy relationship with food.

Pure Agony

It was an agonizing three months. I simply despised sticking to this diet. I don't have incredible willpower so I stayed away from a lot of socializing unless it was my free day. I had to stay focused. Anyway, the results after three months were depressing. At the end of three months I lost about 3 pounds and a little body fat. I looked marginally better in a bathing suit. My "transformation" didn't amount to any more than if I stuck with a sensible diet.

So what happened to me? Of course I blamed myself. Was it the handful of Captain Crunch I had that day? Did I eat too much on my "off" day? Could I have pulled off one more squat? Was I exercising too much?

The Result of My Quest

Did I feel great about myself after three months? To the contrary, my self-esteem was lower than ever before! I was destined to be fat. Why did I bother? You are worthless. You didn't do it. He said I could. I still have loads of cellulite. He said it would go away! It worked for everyone in the magazine. What did I do wrong? Did they ever eat the Captain Crunch like I did? Was that it?

So I guess you can see the problem I have with Phillips. He sets people up with unrealistic goals, shows you how other people achieved miraculous results and says you can achieve them too. When we fail, we blame ourselves.

Within a month of going off the diet I gained back the weight and body fat I lost. The stringent lifestyle was not worth the results.

The concept behind *Body for Life* is great. He emphasizes good nutrition, regular exercise and weight training – a perfect combination. But his stringent tactics and overstated results are not realistic for the average person and it sabotages the credibility of the positive things he says.

It's the Packaging That Counts

Along with the diet best-sellers are the conveniently packaged diet programs. These include pre-packaged portion controlled programs like Jenny Craig; the meal replacement or supplement diets like Slim Fast; and all liquid diets like The Hollywood 48-Hour Miracle Diet.

While there is nothing necessarily wrong with the programs, the concept practices food avoidance instead of food acceptance. The programs don't work unless you make them work. If you have a can of Slim Fast for lunch, you still have to have the willpower to not eat anything else and then maintain control through your "sensible" dinner. If you already have trouble eating too much food, why would you choose to go on a diet that eliminated even more "real" food?

Pre-packaged food programs don't work unless you eat only the rationed boring and expensive foods they give you. You still need willpower not to dive in and raid the refrigerator anyway. These work especially well for desperate people who are short on motivation. They wake up one morning and decide, "Today's the day." They hand over their wallets to the program as their affirmation of dedication, only to fall back to their old habits before the check has cleared.

Temporary liquid diets (emergency diets) claim to cleanse the user of toxins and guarantee weight loss of up to 10 pounds in 2 days. While it is possible you can lose that much, it's not fat loss. It's water and waste loss. Our bodies are 80% water. It's easy to lose weight by extracting water, but that's not the same as losing fat. Go off the diet and except for the benefit of the calories not ingested, you will gain it all back.

The ingredients of these products are ridiculous. The Hollywood 48-Hour Miracle Diet, for example, costs $24.99 at a bargain price. The only ingredients are concentrated fruit juice with added vitamins and minerals. You don't eat anything for 2 days and *voila!* 10 pounds lost! You could do the same thing by eating nothing but apples and grapefruit and taking a vitamin pill.

Dieting the "All Natural" Way

Natural foods *are* better and we should be moving in a natural food direction. The healthier we eat, the better.

But the diet industry has repackaged healthy diet philosophies and turned them into a magic solution to everyone's weight problems. Illusionary people buy these books with the premise of miraculously losing weight and becoming a purist. They can't seem to pass up super-sizing their #5 meal at McDonald's, but their expectation is to read a book and suddenly prefer to live on tofu and wheat germ.

Maximum health diet books used to be written for people who are finding alternative treatments for an illness or are already eating a healthy diet and are seeking a cleaner lifestyle. There aren't enough people in this country falling into the health "extremist" category to warrant the sale of enough book copies to reach the best-seller list.

Weight Watchers International – A Diet You Can Live With

Weight Watchers is by far the most popular and successful weight loss program and with good reason. Weight Watchers uses a common sense, usable philosophy of modifying caloric intake without eliminating any food category. The Weight Watchers program customizes a point plan and allows you to eat whatever you want as long as you stay within your point (calorie) range. If followed, the program works because you must account for everything you eat. Additionally, they provide a support system and a maintenance program to help the successful "losers" keep the pounds off.

While the point system is proclaimed by the public to be easier, counting calories is more educational. Nutrition labeling provides you with portion and calorie values as well as fat, protein and carbohydrate content. There are many comprehensive "value of food" books on the market that itemize the calories and components of food. I think if you are going to "count" anything, you are better off counting calories. Unfortunately, our society will do anything to avoid counting calories and Weight Watchers is well aware of that fact.

The Weight Watcher program's ultimate goal is to help people develop better *lifetime* eating habits, but because some of us perceive it as a "diet," they go into the program with a short-term goal. Some are successful and learn from the program, but many want to lose weight in a hurry so it will be over and they can return to their old eating lifestyles.

Sometimes the support system can fail when a participant doesn't want to own up to a sudden pound gained. They deliberately miss a weekly weigh-in, vow to be extra good the next week and soon stop going. The action creates the on-again, off-again syndrome. "I've got to go back to Weight Watchers" is a common statement made by temporary Weight Watchers winners. Their short-term success indicates that they haven't really learned to stay in control of their food consumption by choice. They want someone else to tell them what to do. They haven't really learned anything in the process.

If you choose Weight Watchers as *your* way to lose weight, you need to plan for a future without Weight Watchers. How are you going to view food going forward? How do you intend to keep the weight off? Don't view Weight Watchers as a temporary diet. Figure out how you are going to work nutrition, moderation and control into your life forever.

Diets Revealed

So what have we learned? Plenty. Most of the recently marketed diet plans that have hit the best-seller lists are using smoke and mirrors brainwashing. They disguise the truth by using unproven theories to convince you that their plan works because of the formula, method or system. The truth? All of them are merely low-calorie diets.

They use points, blocks, percentages, units and windows to obfuscate the truth – anything but the dirty word – CALORIES.

They talk about visions and inner strength and "eat all you want as long as . . . " They rarely mention the dreaded word – WILLPOWER.

It's a shame because along with the illogical bad advice, some of the diets do provide some good advice that could be better communicated.

We are more confused and frustrated than ever. We used to know what "balanced nutrition" was but now, with so many theories and gimmicks, we don't know what to eat, let alone how to eat.

We are avoiding the only thing we know for sure: Whatever we're eating, we're eating too much of it!

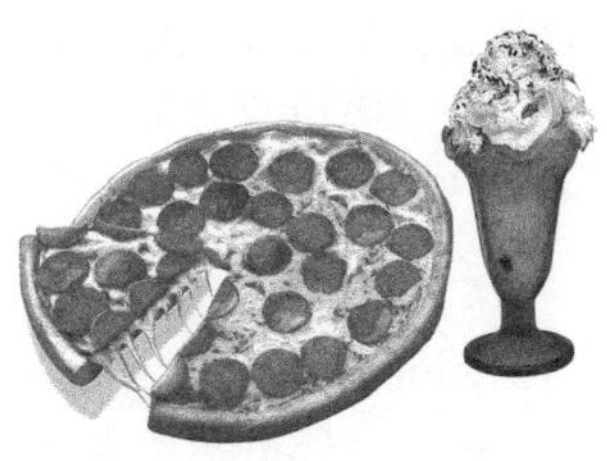

Chapter 6

Gadgets, Gurus and Weight Loss Supplements

Gadgets

Don't you get aggravated every time you watch an infomercial pitching a new exercise aid with totally outlandish claims? "Have the body you always wanted in only 12 minutes a day!" they claim. Then they show a gorgeous, twenty-something athletic instructor using their product, smiling, without sweating, who says, "You can look like this too!"

Give me a break. I'll tell you right now, if you are overweight and out of shape there isn't an exercise contraption in the world that's going to make you look like her. If you completely changed your lifestyle it would take years, not weeks, to achieve that kind of goal. Even then, you're not likely to look like her except in your dreams.

Just Make It Easy

Why do we believe such ridiculous claims? We want a quick fix. We want exercise to be easy and we want results fast. So we spend our hard earned dollars in the hopes of finding the "magic" even though our sensible heads tell us it's not going to happen.

Commercials tell us what we want to hear. Common sense goes out the window and we actually believe because we want to believe. The FTC requires infomercials to offer buyers a 30-day return guarantee. But the likelihood that we will return the product is slim because we were too lazy to actually use the product long enough to challenge the guarantee.

The Best Pick

I'm not saying all exercise products are bad. Traditional cardio machines like treadmills, stair steppers and the like are all good cardio machines. But typically, they aren't the ones pitching the exaggerated hype.

Consumer advocates and exercise physiologists have performed tests to see which of the popular aerobic machines gave the best results. The differences were negligible.

The machines only work as hard as you do. You can burn 1,000 calories on a treadmill or 100; it depends on the intensity and duration of your workout. You determine how well it works by how long, how hard and how often you use the machine.

The real difference, experts say, is in which machine you are most inclined to use. You might burn a few extra calories per 10 minutes on a stair stepper, but if you are more inclined to walk on a treadmill, then a treadmill is a better cardio machine *for you.* A machine only works if you use it. So if you want to invest in a piece of equipment, go for the one you are most likely to use, not the one the infomercials say will give you the best results.

My favorite cardio machine is a treadmill. Almost everyone can walk. It's versatile and suitable for the entire family. You can take a leisurely stroll while watching TV or you can do a five-mile run with Led Zeppelin blaring in your headset. You can walk uphill (a great calorie burner and easier on the knees) and your kids can even use it. I wish I could get my dog on it!

Amazing Abs

There are dozens of abdominal machines and contraptions on the market that say they'll give you the abs you've always wanted. The advertisement might show a fat guy trying to do a sit-up with his head all scrunched up into his chest, sweaty and looking disgusted. Then they show a lean, gorgeous 20-year-old using their hyped machine with six-pack abs. The advertisers lead you to believe that the fat guy is going to turn into the buff kid if he uses the machine. The fat guy could completely overhaul his lifestyle and perform 1,000 repetitions with their gadget every day for two years and, most likely, he still wouldn't have those stylish abs they say you will get in only six weeks.

The Worst of the Worst

My pick for the worst abdominal product is a widely advertised abdominal contraption at a high cost of nearly $100. You sit in this chair and hang your arms over bars and lean forward, back and all around. *"Not only do you tackle all the abdominal area, but it's an aerobic workout as well!"* they say. I tried it and it's the most ridiculous thing I've ever used! Not only did I not feel my abs working, I had to stop after 3 minutes because the back support roller was killing me. And my heart rate didn't increase any more than if I got up to go to the refrigerator.

No matter what abdominal infomercials claim, you cannot spot reduce any area of your body. Working your abs can strengthen the abdominal muscles and help your posture, but it doesn't make you lose fat. You can't turn fat into muscle.

The only way to lose fat is to reduce calories and/or expend calories. Personally, I think the basic floor crunch works better than any of the machines. A properly executed crunch should not put any strain on the neck or back. But since we don't know any better we think we need to rely on a gadget to do the work for us.

The Disclaimers

If you watch the infomercials closely, you will notice tiny writing at the bottom of the commercials or key words used in the dialogue disclosing the bubble bursting reality. You'll see a disclaimer in tiny print that says, "When used in conjunction with a modified diet and exercise program" (of course you'll see results, you're dieting and exercising!) or "claimed results not typical" or "will vary."

I suggest if you are a couch potato, before you go out and spend hundreds of dollars on a piece of equipment you may use as a clothes hanger, put on your walking shoes and take a walk. If you can walk consistently for a month, then go spend the money on a machine. Buying a machine is not going to make you lose weight; using the machine will. If *you* don't do it; it won't get done.

The Gurus

Many products or theories are verified "believable" because they are sponsored or created by professionals. Doctors, athletes, nutritionists, psychologists, models and movie stars are used to validate the products' integrity.

We think the machine must work because they used it and have a great body. This diet theory must work. After all, she's a doctor or he's a nutritionist and they know everything about it. They say it's so, so it must be so.

The talk show psychologist says it's a dysfunctional childhood that has caused me to be fat; I am a weak person, that's why I am fat; I'm an emotional eater, that's why I'm fat; I hate myself, that's why I'm fat. With this admission, you are supposed to look in the mirror, vow to change, snap your fingers and *presto!* You're cured! While much of this may be true, you can't just say it and change it, and maybe it's not even true.

Therapy or Bullying?

I get a lot of flack for saying this but I think some of the popular psychology experts are bullies. They do offer some very good advice, but sometimes it seems they make a person feel terrible about themselves in the process. They might finger point and say, "You know what your problem is?" and proceed to tell them when they don't even know them.

The victim is already feeling inferior because they can't control their eating. I don't think being intimidated by a pompous finger pointer is going to make them feel any better.

How do they really know how you feel? How can they simplify one's psychological need (assuming it is psychological) for food without knowing all the information? How can they sum up the answer with one message? You know what *your* problem is . . . ?

Don't Be Blinded by Authority

I'm not saying the gurus are all crooks, but we shouldn't believe everything we hear just because it's written or said by a "so-called" expert. Barry Sears, the author of *The Zone,* is a good example. His theories are completely unfounded and most of his peers claim his theories have no evidence to support them and his claim that "bad" eicosanoids cause disease is "ridiculous."

Yet, when you read his book, the medical terminology and discussion on the physiological process is so complex, we just assume it's true because we are not educated enough to argue about it. It sounds impressive so we believe it.

Understand that the "experts" are also human. They have the same hopes and dreams as you or me and making money or achieving fame may be their real motivator. It might be an ego thing or maybe they have just inadvertently skewed their research because they want to believe too.

The athlete may not have ever used the product. The doctor may be completely aware of their diet theory's hocus-pocus. They know they can make a lot of money from us because we want to hear what they have to say and we want to believe them. If we weren't buying it, they wouldn't be selling it.

A humorous observation by Charles R. Attwood, M.D., F.A.A.P, author of *A Giant Leap Backwards* is that both Dr. Sears and Dr. Atkins have exceeded the upper limits of weight recommended by federal guidelines. It's like the shoemaker's son that doesn't have shoes.

My Favorite Guru

The flamboyant Richard Simmons is my favorite guru. His emotionally charged, highly marketed diet system has had its share of laughs, but the program is really very good. He uses a common sense approach to losing weight and shows realistic results from real people.

The weight plan works like Weight Watchers but he uses windows instead of points to avoid the dreaded "C" word. But what made his program special are his videos. They are truly motivating even for a seasoned couch potato. He doesn't have lean, muscular women performing strenuous, complicated routines. Instead, his "set" is a living room filled with women of all different sizes from slim to outright obese! The movements are easy and the music is familiar and fun. The message his videos send is powerfully simple: "Look, that woman is fat like me, but she can do it and she's having fun!" What a great motivator for someone who is struggling with self-esteem. He provides methods, guidance and motivation in the privacy of one's home.

He relates to obese people and in the Richard Simmons realm, success isn't measured in a bikini. When you buy his program you're not buying into unrealistic expectations. Richard Simmons is realistic; he went from fat to healthy. He's energized and happy (at least he seems to be). I've got to give Richard Simmons credit. He uses a modified lower calorie, nutritionally balanced diet and exercise program. He focuses on realistic expectations and has packaged it in an irresistible, motivating way.

The Great Weight Loss Supplement Rip-Off

Americans spend billions on vitamin and food supplements, and the pill pushing industry has grown phenomenally in the last 10 years. Some of us are spending hundreds of dollars a month searching for eternal health. Weight loss supplements continue to be the most popular. We are looking for a "magic" pill that will make us thinner and healthier. What could be easier?

My Marketing Idea

If I had the money, I could package a sugar pill and call it "Unlimited Energy in a Bottle" and sell it to a million people on the Internet. I could repackage Ex-lax, call it "Coloclens," and claim you'll lose 3 pounds overnight or your money back. I don't need approval from the FDA. All I need is a buyer. I can't outright lie, but I can make the product convincing even while disclosing the truth.

You hear the disclosures on the infomercials. "Research *suggests*," is one ambiguous standby. Or, "clinically proven to *possibly* make you lose weight." Unfortunately, "clinically proven" is all we hear. The "possibly" part we don't hear, either consciously or unconsciously. After all, we want to believe it.

The Winners of the Secretly Disguised

A crazy infomercial I saw the other day proclaimed their fat sucking pill would absorb 20 grams of fat. If taken three times a day, it could absorb over 500 calories. *"We all know we aren't going to change our lifestyles, so here is a way to lose all the weight you want without dieting – guaranteed!"* I perked up on this one! They actually used real numbers. The commercial came right out and stated how many calories you could save a day taking this miracle pill.

But wait, what's this? While viewing the testimonials I see a tiny disclosure: "Modified diet and exercise *required* to lose weight." Wait a minute! If you are eliminating 500 calories a day (I don't want to think how it is eliminated) aren't you going to lose a pound a week (one pound = 3500 calories) without doing anything else?

But the winning phrase in the category of the secretly disguised is: "One hundred percent of the people who use this product *might* see results." Sound impressive? I could make that statement with anything. Buy a lottery ticket and you *might* win a million dollars!

A Dangerous Best-Seller

Ephedra (also known as ma huang or ephedrine) is one of the most popular diet drugs on the market today. Ephedra is marketed under numerous names; the most widely advertised is Metabolife, Xenadrine and Hydroxycuts. The "all natural" substance is now found in numerous weight loss products typically with the name in part being "thermo" something.

There is some proof that ephedra can increase metabolism causing your body to burn more calories. It also suppresses appetite and increases energy. While ephedra may be proven to increase metabolism somewhat, the appetite suppressant factor is the real weight loss magic. I've taken ephedra and find the effects similar to "speeding."

Ephedra manufacturers say it is safe when taken as directed, but some people have had bad experiences with the herbal drug and the FDA is watching closely. *U.S. News & World Report* stated that an attorney in California is suing the makers of one highly marketed ephedra product on behalf of 13 clients who claim to have suffered brain damage, seizures and possibly even death after taking the drug. And those statistics are growing. Another report claims that the FDA believes that ephedra may be related to more than 50 deaths.

If you search the Internet, you will find dozen of web sites advertising ephedra products. You will also find dozens of law office web sites offering their services to sue manufacturers for health damages as a result of ephedra.

We've been bamboozled into believing that because the wonder product is "natural," the ingredients are safe. The conclusion is pretty stupid when you consider the effects of marijuana, peyote or other "all-natural" substances.

My Harrowing Ephedra Experience

I had adverse effects while taking ephedra. I'm the type of person who gets jittery taking an antihistamine. Taking ephedra for me was like taking *five times* the dose of an antihistamine. In the initial hours after taking the drug I felt energetic and almost euphoric. I didn't have much of an appetite and the first few hours of the day were wonderful.

As the day went on, however, I began to get spacey, nervous and irritable. The unsettling feeling made me want to eat even though I wasn't really hungry. I wanted something, but I couldn't figure out what. I was going crazy! I just wanted to feel normal again. My heart was racing and I wanted to tear my hair out! I ended up eating a lot at the end of the day as I was coming "down" from the drug's effects.

Even when I stopped taking the recommended third dose for the day, I couldn't get to sleep at night. Personally, I found the side effects of ephedra more powerful than chemical "speed." I kept this up for about a week. I started to get paranoid and depressed. I haven't taken it since.

Do You Want to Risk It?

Ephedra is like an all-natural "speed." It has potentially dangerous side effects. If you do lose weight, the only way you are going to keep it off is by continuously taking the drug. Even so, with continued use, you will build up a tolerance to its effectiveness. Before you buy into the ephedra fad, consider if taking drugs is the way you want to lose weight. Is the short-term possible weight loss worth risking your health?

The Distant Runner-ups

Some other "all-natural," supposedly safe supplements are pyruvate, chromium, chitosol, synephrine, kava kava and others. While research "suggests" some of the supplements may produce thermogenic or other weight loss abilities, the actual effectiveness is disappointing, to say the least. Most are appetite suppressants and some may produce negative side effects. They typically work by making you feel like you are about to give a speech or have an anxiety attack. Is that how you want to feel?

The Disappointing Bottom Line

Don't trust the hype. If you want to find out the truth behind the product you want to try, bypass the TV and the commercial web sites with their biased opinions. Research medically documented opinions and research findings. Let's face it, if the pill really worked, we'd know about it. It would be groundbreaking, front-page news.

Is There Magic in RX?

There are some prescribed products that claim to reduce the appetite. If you are seriously overweight your doctor might prescribe this drug for you. They're advertised as an appetite suppressant that can assist someone who is serious about losing weight. Since the U.S. Food and Drug Administration monitors the drug, the claims are realistic and the potential side effects are disclosed. Even so, I can't help but remember Phen-fen.

The Rule: Caveat Emptor

Some people are spending over $100 a month or more on diet and health supplements (like I did). While they may not be totally worthless, the effectiveness of the product needs to be weighed against the money spent and the unknown health risks. If you aren't serious about losing weight and willing to do the other basic requirements for weight loss, diet aids aren't going to help at all.

Adding to the unsubstantiated claims of these products is the inflated value of highly marketed products versus generic or less advertised products. Some of the price differences are dramatic. You can spend almost twice as much for a name brand as a generic with the same ingredients. Also, dosage size can be deceiving. Some pills may appear cheaper but you may need two pills instead of one to equal the same level of effectiveness. One pill can't do more than another if they both have the same ingredients.

Two years ago I was taking nearly every one of these "all-natural" weight loss supplements with no results except for a hole in my pocket. I haven't taken any of these supplements in over two years and I weigh the same and have maintained the same body fat level. I wish I had all the money I spent. I could go to the Bahamas for a vacation.

Diets, Gadgets, Gurus and Weight Loss Supplements

What Have We Learned?

We can simplify all of the information in a few words:

Diets

All diets require you to eat fewer calories. Most require that you not only eat fewer calories, but also restrict, forbid or limit some category of food – usually the food you love most. No matter how scientific it sounds it's all about the calorie. You have to have willpower not to eat the extra calories. Don't believe otherwise. It's the same concept we've been using for years, just repackaged into moneymaking, brainwashing schemes.

Gadgets

Exercise machines and gadgets can help you expend calories. All cardio activity burns about the same amount of calories. Regardless, you only reduce calories at a rate your body is expending calories. If you burn more calories, it's because you are working harder, not the machine.

You can't burn any calories if you don't use it.

Gurus

Don't be quick to look up to people who are so-called experts. Don't be vulnerable to their power. Listen to their words, but don't be blinded by their authority. Above all do not consider them better than you or necessarily trustworthy. Educate yourself. Become your own guru.

Weight Loss Supplements

While there may be clinical research that suggests some of the "miracle pills" might stimulate weight loss, results will only be realized if you also include diet and exercise. Most supplements are expensive and some are downright dangerous. Don't waste your money or risk your health.

There are no miracles. Accept it. Put it all behind you.

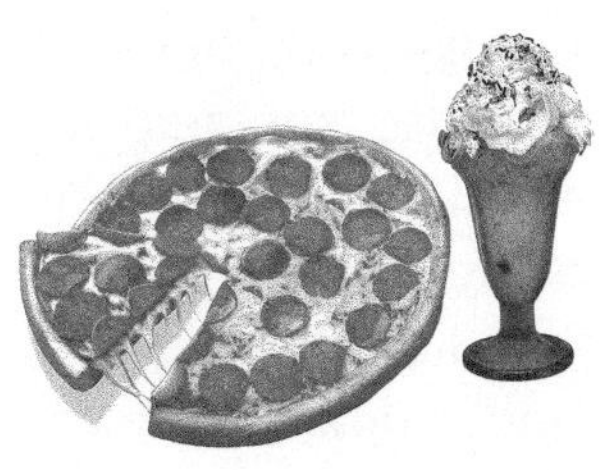

Chapter 7

9 Steps to The NEW You

The diet industry has developed a thousand ways to lose weight and we're still not losing weight. They told us they had *the* answer but it wasn't there. So if a diet, gadget or supplement isn't the answer, then what *is* the answer?

You can't find your answer until you know your problem – and usually your weight issues are comprised of more than one problem. The 9 Steps to The NEW You will help you discover *your* problem and find *your* answer.

Face it. The only way to lose weight and be healthy is to eat a moderate diet and get regular exercise. I know you're telling yourself, "But I've tried eating healthy and exercising and it's too hard! I can't do it!" Yes you can but our minds and emotions are preventing us from doing it. And usually there is more than one reason why they are getting in the way of our ability to succeed.

You can live a healthy lifestyle free from weight issues and it's easy once you get rid of the negative feelings and actions that are preventing you from doing it. You *can* learn to enjoy food, all food, without sacrifice and regret.

The NEW You involves a new way of thinking, a new way of listening and a new way of behaving. I developed the concept as a result of my own changes. While I was able to keep my weight down, it wasn't until I changed my way of thinking and listening that I overcame my problem.

The 9 Step concept begins with an analysis of our environment and how it has negatively changed our ability to live a healthier lifestyle. Its purpose is to help you evaluate and explain why *you* have developed negative emotions about food and how it has impacted how you feel about yourself. You have to find the cause(s) of your problem in order to find your answer. You have to believe you can change your behaviors and you have to truly want to change.

Once you accomplish this, *then* you can move on to the actual changes in your lifestyle that will make you successful. If you can change the way you think and listen, implementing healthy behaviors will be easy.

9 Steps for Change

The path we'll take for the 9 Steps To The NEW You is broken down into three parts. The components and purpose of the three parts will help you to figure out how each may have affected your ability to succeed. You will be able to discover which of the three areas negatively affect you most and it will be the foundation for your change. These are the 9 Steps you will follow:

Part I

A New Way of Thinking

Steps 1 through 4 analyze the emotional side of your problem.

Step 1 Overcoming Your Negative Environment
Step 2 Identify and Stop Blame and Denial
Step 3 Accept Realities and Move On
Step 4 Getting Ready for Change

Part II

A New Way of Listening

Steps 5 and 6 discuss how the impact of dieting and food labeling have affected our ability to know what our body wants and needs. With new listening skills you will learn to trust yourself with food again.

Step 5 Listen to Your Body, Not Your Mind
Step 6 Identify and Conquer Bad Habits

Part III

A New Way of Behaving (The NEW You)

With a new emotional and mental approach to your problem, you will be ready to successfully implement the physical actions that will change your life – to become a NEW You!

Step 7 Nutrition for The NEW You
Step 8 Exercise for The NEW You
Step 9 Weight Training for The NEW You

As you learn about the 9 Steps remember that you might not see your problem in some of the steps. Remember, we all don't have the same problem. Maybe you don't have mirror obsession, but you have bad habits you need to overcome. Maybe you are obsessed with food, but maybe it's just because you are confused. The purpose is self-discovery – to find yourself within these pages.

Be open-minded. You may find issues you hadn't realized – issues that are your real problem. More than likely, you will find you have a combination of issues – the way you think, listen and behave – that are preventing you from being successful. As I said, if you have all the pieces of your puzzle, you will be on the right path to success. Discovering them is the key.

Let's begin our journey to the NEW You.

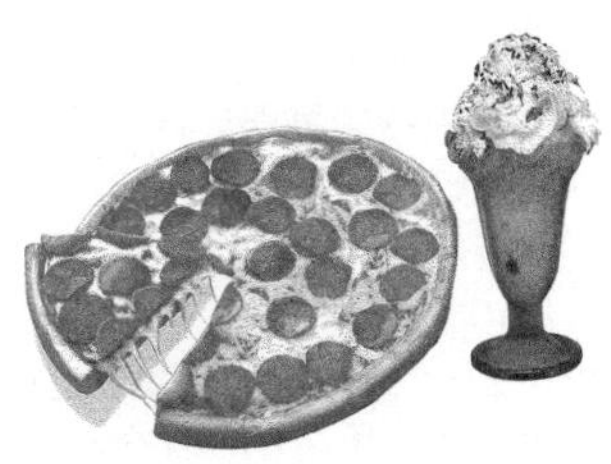

Part I
A New Way of Thinking

How we think about food, ourselves and its impact on our weight has been negatively affected by our environment. We have lost sight of reality when it comes to our expectations of how our body can look. We're analyzing food too much and it's causing a negative emotional reaction to food rather than a natural, biological need for food. Meanwhile food is more readily available; unfortunately the most readily available is fattening and nearly void of nutrition.

The impact of our inability to reach physical expectations and our preoccupation with food has caused us to feel poorly about ourselves. We have gone into denial and look to blame something else. For some of us, our feeling of self-worth revolves around how we look and how food is controlling us. We feel weak, powerless and unworthy. We don't think we can change. We really don't *want* to change. Or maybe we are afraid of change.

Changing how we view ourselves, food and our attitudes about healthy living will give you a foundation for success.

Spend some time being truthful with yourself. Often we are not focusing on the real reasons we are overweight. Why do you think you eat too much? Do you feel good about who you are? Do you make excuses for yourself? Are you in denial? Do you ever get jealous of someone who looks better, physically, than you? Do you ever feel inferior to someone simply because they have a better body than you? Are you comfortable in your own body? Why *are* you adverse to exercise? Are you happy with your current lifestyle? Do you feel capable of change? Can you see yourself being a healthy, active person?

Think about why you have weight issues. If your immediate answer is an excuse, then dig deeper and find a better answer. Excuses will not get you where you want to be. First, identify and admit your problems. Then you can try to solve them.

The first four steps to achieving success have to do with how we view our situation, our food and ourselves. The objective is to mentally prepare you for a lifestyle change.

I already (hopefully) convinced you that there is no magic to diets, pills and products. Below are listed the four steps in the "thinking" strategy.

Step 1

Overcoming Our Negative Environment

Examine why you might have developed negative thinking about your lifestyle and yourself;

Step 2

Identify and Stop Blame and Denial

Explore what happened to you as a result of your negative thinking. How to identify blame and denial tactics to overcome them;

Step 3

Accept Realities and Move On

Change your negative thinking by learning and accepting the unchangeable realities about your expectations so you can move forward in a more positive direction;

Step 4

Getting Ready For Change

Convince yourself that you can change. You have to believe that living a healthy lifestyle is not hard and is something you want to do and not something you have to do.

With your new way of thinking, you can prepare yourself to implement the positive changes in your life that will lead to A NEW You.

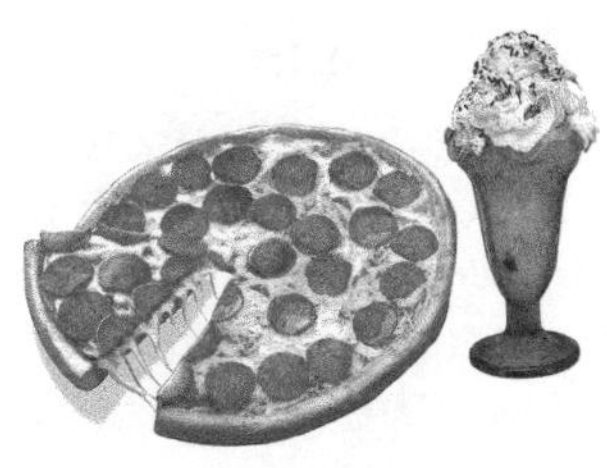

Chapter 8

STEP 1
Overcoming Our Negative Environment

Today's environment has created negative attitudes regarding our relationship with food and ourselves. The media is dictating the definition of beauty and health. Food is readily available, widely advertised and void of good nutrition, and the diet industry is making us believe the unbelievable. The medical community is constantly changing its definition of healthy foods and our lives are so stressed out we can't seem to focus on what our bodies need.

Step 1 will address how the following issues have adversely affected our thinking.

- Identifying the Media's Bogus View of Beauty
- How Our Lifestyles Have Changed Our Eating Habits
- How Our Environment Has Adversely Affected Our Relationship With Food
- How Food and Expectations Impact How We Feel About Ourselves

Exploring the problems of our environment might help you to understand your negative attitudes and emotions towards food and yourself.

Identifying the Media's Bogus View of Beauty

The media defines beauty. Television, movies, magazines, runways and catalogs all dictate the definition of what's "beautiful" today. Surely Jayne Mansfield or Marilyn Monroe would be considered "cows" by today's media. They wouldn't be able to get a job. You can just see the tabloids: "Monroe to get walking papers on the set of *Some Like It Hot* unless she loses 25 pounds!" Think of the classic photo where the air is blowing up her dress. Would she have looked better with less meat on her bones? Of course not!

What we thought was beautiful even 10 years ago in a woman's body is now considered "piggish." I saw an article that viewed three young stars and their "transformation" from just five years ago. They were slim to begin with, but now they are emaciated. The realistic world calls them "lollipop heads" because they are so skinny their heads look too big for their bodies. Why would anyone try to look like that? Yet, Hollywood is embracing this new look and it has influenced society's view of the "ideal" woman.

The new "vogue" style has placed more demands on us to adjust our bodies to follow the trend. Since most of us could never reach the goal we give up and conclude, "If I can't be thin, I might as well give up and be fat! If being a healthy size 12 isn't good enough, why bother!"

The Obstacles Get Harder

Not only are women expected to be thin, but now we are also expected to be strong. Six pack abs and bulging muscles are displayed as feminine and desirable. It certainly isn't natural for a woman's body to look like that. I don't think it's attractive, do you? Don't get me wrong; there is nothing wrong with a well-shaped, toned body but we are taking it to the extremes.

Yet, at times I felt inferior to these women even though I knew better. Now, not only are they thin, some of them are spending hours in the gym sculpting their genetically blessed bodies to raise the bar even higher. I incorrectly conclude they are stronger and better than me; I'm not disciplined like they are.

Boobs, Belly Buttons and Booties

When we used to think of beauty we thought of a pretty smile, shining hair, a curvy figure or shapely legs. In today's highly sexual environment it's all about the boobs, the belly buttons and the booties. You don't have to be facially attractive anymore; as long as you've got the 3 B's you are envied and adored.

But usually the boobs are fake, the bellies are emaciated and the booties are airbrushed. So what makes a size 2 body so attractive to men? Why is it in the old days men liked a little meat on the bones but today drool over waifs?

It's because with modern cosmetic surgery, we are able to redefine the definition of symmetry. Hollywood idols can diet themselves down to near anorexia and then slap on a pair of double D's. They look like they are going to fall over. Personally, I think the new idea of symmetry looks ridiculous but as long as men can drool over cleavage, they don't need to look at anything else.

Yet we feel less of a woman because our breasts (if we had much to start with) are sagging after nursing our kids. Our bellies are stretched out and scarred from childbirth and our booties are only seen in the most unflattering light. While the "perfect" people put themselves first, the average woman's personal needs are last on her overwhelming list of things to do. And the $3,000 they had saved up for the cosmetic surgery of their dreams just went to pay the roofing bill.

Reality Tells a Different Story

But we think we should look like them. We cover our bodies and tell ourselves we are fat, ugly and unworthy. Unfortunately we've gotten so self-conscious of our bodies we hide ourselves, embarrassed by our imperfections.

Look around you. Look at the real world. When I go the beach, I don't see the gorgeous tanned beauties roller-blading down the boardwalk. What I see are ordinary people – all shapes and sizes. Rarely do I see a woman that looks even close to what I see on TV or in magazines.

We place the unrealistic expectation on ourselves. Others typically don't view a thin person as an ideal figure. A study published in the *International Journal of Eating Disorders* had participants of different ages evaluate drawings of people of varying sizes and rate their attractiveness. The volunteers judged people in the midrange of fatness to be the most socially acceptable, while those who were very thin or obese did not fare as well. So why do we even want to achieve such an unrealistic look?

Hiding Limits Activity

Some of us are so embarrassed by our perceived unattractive bodies that we don't dare show them to anyone. We consider our imperfections ugly and disgusting so we hide them in embarrassment. When we take our clothes off we turn the lights out because we feel our bodies are flawed, unlike the images we see in the media. We wear oversized unrevealing clothes because we don't want anyone to see our imperfections.

Participating in activities with noticeable body movement or that require little clothing are limited. We don't go in the pool because we'd have to wear a bathing suit. We don't go to a gym or take an aerobics class because we might have to show too much of ourselves in public. Why does it matter so much? Why can't we just do what we want without feeling judged by our appearance?

Our Negative Attitude Exacerbates the Problem

Our "imperfect" facial features don't prevent us from feeling worthy of respect or love, yet many of us don't feel the same way when it comes to our bodies. Like our facial features, every "body" is different and unique. We don't wear a bag over our head to hide a big nose, but we can hide our bodies, and we do.

Hiding our body allows us to ignore what's happening under there and can contribute to obesity. Once you start hiding your figure, it's easier to gain more weight. Why? Because you have accepted the fact that no one is going to see your body. So if you are going to hide it anyway, what's another 10 pounds? It's easier today with all the casual dressing; elastic-waist pants with flowing tunics; long sweaters over leggings; jumpers; or sweat pants. We can hide it so easily. Remember Ethel Mertz from *I Love Lucy?* She was robust, but she still wore shirtdresses with cinched waists. Put *that* on every morning (with a girdle) and you'd think twice about that Krispy Kreme donut!

Baby Bulge Blues

When women get pregnant, many quickly go down the "body hiding" path. They have the baby, put themselves second and hide their body under their maternity tent. They keep wearing their tent during postpartum because it's easier to wear the tent than to put themselves first and work at getting their figure back.

I've observed that post-baby women who are quick to put on their jeans (maybe with the button undone at first) are more likely to get down to their pre-pregnancy weight than those that continue to wear their pregnancy clothes. When you're wearing the maternity tent who's to notice – including you!

Once you get used to wearing the tent, it's hard to go back. If you are unhappy with your body and want to change, the first thing you need to do is get out of the tent. Put those jeans on you can't get over your butt and look in the mirror. Buy a pair of new jeans that fit (not too loose) and make your first goal not to outgrow those pants. Make your second goal to fit back into the first pair.

Can Society Change Its View of the Ideal?

Just like clothing, being ultra thin is a fashion trend. It's not the definition of true beauty. Society can change the definition of the "ideal." Recently I picked up a fashion magazine at the hairdressers and was admiring the clothes when it occurred to me that the models weren't waifs! It's not that they were obese, but they were about a size 10-14, not a size 1-4. We are so used to seeing non-skinny women portrayed with poor lighting, bad clothes and no make-up as seen in the "before" pictures. Given the same environmental conditions as Victoria's Secret models, these larger models look beautiful even in their underwear! I'm serious! It was refreshing, unique, exciting!

While it's unrealistic for the average woman to be a size 2, it is realistic for an average woman to achieve a healthy size 10 or 12. If the media allowed the same environmental conditions as the thin people emulated, we could change the look of the ideal, beautiful woman.

The Truth About Cellulite – We All Have It

I was at the gym observing a rather unique woman. She was bony with hunks of muscle (like Popeye). She had a manly V-shape back and completely defined arms. Her upper body was large, yet she looked emaciated. She didn't look like a body builder because she was too skinny. She didn't look athletic because she didn't look healthy. I was viewing her from the treadmill and I could only see her from the waist up. Later, I got a full view of her.

She was standing in front of a mirror examining her legs. As thin as she was, she still had a little meat and cellulite on her thighs. I noticed she gave a disappointed look as she went back to her lifting.

I felt sorry for her for I've been there too. She probably starves herself and spends countless hours in the gym trying to reduce her body fat to unrealistic levels, only to be disappointed by her failure to achieve the goal of having rock hard, cellulite-free thighs.

Everyone talks about cellulite today. I don't remember anyone talking about it a generation ago. We keep hearing that cellulite is the result of excess fat, poor diet and not enough hydration. Everyone says if you just do this or that it will go away.

Well it doesn't!

I have tried everything to control my cellulite, even expensive cellulite treatments (what a waste of money *that* was). And the older I get, the worse it gets. I see loads of cellulite at the gym. From what I observe, it doesn't really matter what size you are. I've seen very athletic women with little body fat have more cellulite than a woman who is 20 pounds overweight and 10 years older.

Nearly every woman over the age of 30 has at least a little cellulite, but we are expected not to have it. You don't see cellulite on models and actresses. It's not because most don't have it but because media pictures make sure they get rid of it. They camouflage the cellulite by soft lighting and airbrushing, if necessary. Even at the ESPN Hawaiian Tropic model contest, I noticed a few bumps and jiggles. The contest was viewed in outdoor lighting (dreadful for exposing cellulite) instead of flattering photographic lighting.

Embracing Imperfection

Wouldn't it be great if the eighteenth century's view of the ideal woman became our ideal again? Like the Rubenesque nude paintings that show the rounded stomach, the ample butt, the milky white skin.

And since we don't have a cure for cellulite, why don't we just embrace it! Smooth texture out, dimpled texture in! Why not?

Wouldn't that take the pressure off of women! So why don't *you* take the pressure off yourself? You don't have to be perfect even if you think society says you do. Consider your so-called imperfections as an attribute of your individuality.

How Our Lifestyles Have Changed Our Eating Habits

Our lifestyles have changed dramatically over the past decade. We have created an environment that makes it easier to neglect our bodies and live unhealthy lifestyles.

Women who are in the throes of raising children suffer the most. Many are stressed out and have little time for themselves. Many women are working and still have the demands at home. And for many the demands at home have gotten worse. We feel guilty not spending enough time with our children so we spend a good chunk of our precious leisure time with our kids. Unfortunately, the time spent with children today revolves around sitting on ball field bleachers *watching them play* instead of *playing with them.*

What Happened to Dinnertime?

Dinnertime has really changed. Because we're not home enough, we don't prepare healthy meals. We rely on fast food, cheap restaurants and processed store bought dinners. If neither Mom nor Dad has time to prepare dinner, what's everyone going to eat? And let's not forget, once we're home we have to run out a half hour later to Ashley's dance class.

Many families don't spend many dinners together. Kids snub their noses at good home-cooked meals and, for the most part, we give in to them. When I was growing up, I can remember the dreaded liver, onion and beet night. I hated these foods and would spit them in my napkin while Mom wasn't looking. My parents didn't cater to my food wishes. You always had to eat your vegetables and you had two choices for dinner: take it or leave it. I eventually learned to eat foods I didn't think I liked because I didn't really have a choice.

Reliance on fattening, highly processed food results in high calories and unhealthy eating for both adults and children. Dinner, especially, should be a time for good food and togetherness.

Our busy lifestyles make it difficult to have healthy meals, but it shouldn't be an excuse. There are ways to remedy the situation. Our environment makes it harder, but it can be done – it should be done. When you convince yourself it's not a hopeless situation, you'll find it's really pretty easy. You'll want to do it.

Food Is Readily Available

Today our social environment is based on food – great food and lots of it. It's common for someone to have a party that can last four hours or more where the only theme is food and drink. I go to these parties and all I do is eat and drink and socialize. At least in the '70's I could stop and have a cigarette. The events are feeding frenzies. Usually everyone brings their favorite hors d'oeuvre or gooey dessert in addition to whatever catered meal is provided. It's sinful!

It takes a lot of willpower not to overeat at these events. That in itself is not so bad, but the frequency has escalated. Some of us treat nearly every meal as a special occasion. It's our entertainment! If food continues to be an overwhelming part of our culture, we have to do something to control our eating. It makes it harder, but we can't use it as an excuse. We have to learn to control our eating even when food is abundant. It shouldn't matter how much food is available; when you've had enough you need to stop eating!

Losing Weight for the Good of the Country

Does that sound absurd? It shouldn't. Whole books have been written on the subject, including the seminal work by Frances Lappe, *Diet for a Small Planet.*

You might not want to hear this but if you are obese, you are a financial burden to this country. The inability to be thin is not an excuse to live an unhealthy lifestyle. Maybe you have a genetic predisposition to gain weight and maybe you have a high tolerance for large quantities of food. Maybe you love food more than the next person. But you can still maintain a moderately healthy lifestyle by eating nutritious foods along with the goodies and getting regular exercise. The reality is most people who have severe weight problems are not even trying to live a healthy lifestyle.

If you can't eat healthier foods and exercise for yourself, then do it as your social responsibility.

Health care costs are out of control. The collective medical costs for those who neglect their bodies exceed the medical cost of the nation's smokers. Obesity often leads to considerably more health problems, including major illnesses like heart disease, diabetes and cancer and minor illnesses like knee problems and sleep apnea as well as stress, depression and other psychological problems. Expensive health care is something we all pay for.

According to recent government figures, 27 percent of American adults are obese. Another 34 percent are overweight. Even more alarming is the recent data (from 1999) reporting that 13 percent of children ages 6-11 are overweight, and 14 percent of children ages 12-19 are overweight. The Surgeon General cites in his February 2002 report on the health of the nation, "If the situation [overweight Americans] is not reversed, it could wipe out the gains we have made in areas such as heart disease, diabetes, several types of cancer and other chronic problems."

It is hard to lose weight and some of us struggle more than others. It's an effort to get up and take a walk when the couch is so comfortable or we just don't feel like it. But, if your weight is contributing to your health problems and you are not doing anything about it, then shame on you!

We remedy many preventable health conditions not with a change in lifestyle, but with pills, surgeries and therapies at a very expensive cost to society. Recent research finds that not only can regular exercise and a healthy, moderate diet control Type II diabetes, but also may actually *prevent* the onset in some cases. This is huge news. If diabetes is indeed preventable by a healthy lifestyle, think of the health care dollars saved and, more importantly, the lives saved and improved.

Another study suggests that three quarters of Type II diabetics admit they aren't following their doctor's orders to eat healthier and exercise. Now researchers have invented a new pill that will help control it for you. While this may be beneficial, it only discourages the unmotivated diabetic from doing anything to change their lifestyle.

Taking Responsibility

The recent Surgeon General's report also points out that weighing too much is the biggest cause of preventable deaths in this country, second only to tobacco. Recent lawsuits have taken responsibility off of smokers and heaped it on tobacco companies. Can't the same case be made against donut shops, snack food makers and fast food restaurants? They all sell products that we know aren't good for us and can cause adverse health effects if not consumed in moderation.

We take the position that tobacco companies are luring children into smoking by using a camel caricature in their advertisements, yet fast food restaurants are bribing children with toys in marketed kids meals! What message is that sending: Hey kids, bypass the chicken and broccoli and bring the family to our high calorie, nutritionally challenged restaurant! We'll even give you a toy if you do!

With the obesity rate high and still climbing, food abuse is a serious factor in our society's health and the nation's wealth. In fact, a recent ABC news sound bite reported suing food companies, especially fast food and vending machine companies, for one's obesity is possible. "There is a movement afoot to do something about the obesity problem, not just as a visual blight but to see it in terms of costs," says John Banzhaf, a George Washington University Law School professor.

While I vehemently oppose slapping the responsibility on others for our weight problems, I do think it's time for our government to provide an incentive to restaurants for providing healthier options like densely nutritious vegetables and lean proteins. How inconvenient would it be for a fast food restaurant to offer a side of steamed broccoli? At least then the public has an option to choose. But, if the public isn't asking for it, the restaurants aren't selling it. If public demand can't influence restaurants, then the government will ultimately have to for our own sake.

So What's Our Option?

We can choose to eat some bad food or a lot of bad food. We can choose to drink two glasses of wine a week, a half-gallon of scotch or none at all. And, believe it or not, you can also choose to have one cigarette a week, a pack a day, or none at all.

We have to stop using our environmental situation as an excuse for our weight problems. When I look at someone who is irresponsibly overweight, I am saddened that they don't care enough about themselves or their loved ones to want to live a healthy life, at any cost. If you are obese, not only are you a burden on society's pocketbook, you run a higher risk of becoming a disabling burden to your family. Or your family may have to face the unnecessary suffering of your premature death. Being obese and not doing anything about it is a slow suicide. Do something about it.

How Our Environment Has Negatively Affected Our Relationship with Food

We think too much about food. Food talk is everywhere about us. It's on talk shows, books, articles and products. Every other day there is a new study claiming this food is good for you, this one is bad. The next thing you know, you hear a sound bite of news information reversing the findings to claim that the good food is now bad for you and the bad food is now good for you. We're starting to go around in circles. Likewise, eating and exercising has been narrowed down to scientific formulas and the new solution changes with the next book, study or product.

We are so overly focused on what we should be doing, we are getting more resistant to do it. We have become a nation totally obsessed with it all and it's doing more harm than good. We're either getting fatter and lazier or we're becoming totally committed to strict dieting and excessive exercising. Either way we are obsessing and are losing sight of reality.

We love food and we hate food. This food is "bad" and that food is "good." We want food, but we can't have food. Are we being good with food today? Or are we being bad with food today? The labeling of food is causing us to have an unhealthy relationship with food.

Is Food Your Enemy or Your Friend?

I used to wonder how people could say, "I'm not hungry anymore" when they are in front of a table full of food. Or take just a slice of cake and be satisfied. I used to think my problem was that I didn't have a turn-off button. I could eat and eat and not really get full. In reality, I would get stuffed to the point of feeling sick and only then would I stop eating.

If you have eaten more calories than you needed in a day, do you go to bed at night feeling like you've done something wrong? As you lie there with the Twinkies gurgling in your stomach, does a part of you blame yourself? Do you feel guilty? Do you feel out of control? More importantly, how many nights are you going to bed feeling like this?

I know if I have a bad day, a day when I don't feel good about myself, or am upset about something, that's when I am weakest. That's when I bake a cake and eat it till I'm ready to explode.

The PMS Friend or Foe Battle

A good example of unfriendly eating is PMS eating. We already feel crappy about ourselves so do we turn to food to make ourselves feel better? Or to make ourselves feel worse? Why do we choose to wallow in our misery by making ourselves even more miserable?

I don't know why when we feel so bad we act in ways that make us feel even worse, instead of doing something that makes us feel better. While food is something to be enjoyed, when you emotionally eat food is the enemy. We know it's the enemy when we are rummaging through the kids' Halloween candy. We can't seem to stop ourselves even though we know it's going to hurt us.

Are You Being Bad or Are You Being Good?

What is your indulgence limit? What amount of food consumption upsets you? Is it a handful or two of chips you didn't need before dinner; is it eating three servings of cookies on your way home from the grocery store; or is it eating a large cheese steak and fries with an entire pie for a chaser?

It's relative. There is no magic calculation of what is okay and what is "bad." We all have to eat. How much or what we eat is a big variable. Forget about the repercussions on the scale; think about how you feel after you eat. Do you know you eat more than you need? Do you eat with regrets? Do you eat until you're sick to your stomach? How bad are you?

The definition of overeating is different for every person. What does it mean to be satisfied? I'd read articles that would tell me to stop eating when I was full. What was "full?" To me, being satisfied was the feeling if I ate one more bite I would explode. "Yeah, now I'm satisfied." How come I couldn't just eat like "normal" people? Then again, how much does a "normal" person eat?

Bad for me at age 18 was hanging out at Jack in the Box with my best friend eating half a dozen tacos, a slew of onion rings and a pony 8-pack of Miller beer.

Bad for me at age 25 was trying to make myself throw up after eating just one piece of pizza.

Bad for me at 31 was leaving the house Sunday morning for take-out breakfast at McDonald's, but first swinging by the Dunkin Donuts and picking up a dozen sinkers. So after an Egg McMuffin, hash browns and pancakes, I'd stuff myself with four or five donuts and only then was I "satisfied." "Are you satisfied now? You pig! God, I feel sick. Why did I do that? What was I thinking? Ugh! I hate myself." Yeah, that was bad.

Bad for me at 42 is having a scone on Sunday morning with my eggs and wheat toast. Okay, maybe I buy one more than I need. With a hot cup of fresh coffee and a morning jazz station lulling in the background, I eat the first one, savoring every morsel. I enjoy being bad. I deserve it. It's a great feeling.

Then, after I eat the first one, I look at the second. Am I full? Am I satisfied? Oh, heck, the moment was over too soon. I start to eat the second one and about halfway through I think to myself, "Why am I eating this? If I eat any more I'm not going to have this great feeling inside me that I feel right now. It will ruin it!" I quickly toss it in the trash (i.e., give it to the dog). It's done, it's over. I was bad, but not that bad. I enjoyed my "badness." If I had finished the second one (and at that point, I could have probably had two more) it wouldn't have been fun anymore. I would have had regrets.

Bad Is Relative

Being "bad" is relative to the person or attitude in question. Don't we all wonder what everyone else "really" eats? We always assume that if we see a thin person take second helpings they must be lucky and have a high metabolism. If we see a fat person pick at dinner and refuse dessert we feel sorry for them. They must have a slow metabolism. But how much do both of these people *really* eat? Is it too little or too much? When we saw them eat, were they being "good" or being "bad"? Was it normal for them?

I Eat, Therefore I'm Fat

We can never be happy eating just enough. It's either way too much or way too little. We're either dieting or binge eating. There is no happy medium any more.

We seem to either reward ourselves with a pint of Haagen Dazs or punish ourselves with a cup of cottage cheese. You feel guilty when you indulge and deprived when you don't.

It's gotten worse with all the fad diets and so-called "good" foods and "bad" foods. Nowadays, even a carrot or an apple can be considered a "no" food. We are receiving mixed messages from all around us. Low fat, high fat, no carb, high carb, all natural, vegetarian, light, cancer causing, cancer preventing, the list goes on and on. We are dazed and confused when it comes to fighting the battle of the bulge. The more we obsess, the more we are possessed.

The more pressure we put on ourselves to eat a certain way, the more deprived and the more out of control we are. We feel sorry for ourselves.

No matter what you eat, it will be on some diet's or doctor's taboo list and the list is ongoing and ever changing. It has gotten to the point that if you tried to find something that wasn't "bad" for you, you really couldn't eat at all!

It used to be that if you ate a big piece of cake or had a double cheeseburger and a large fry, you'd think to yourself, "I shouldn't eat this." Now, you can't have bread, potatoes, meat, fat, sugar, corn, peas, carrots, fruits, I mean what's left! How can you *not* become disillusioned and frustrated? If you believe all this stuff, no wonder you are having problems coping with food.

We have so many experts telling us what to do and what not to do our heads are spinning! The only conclusion one comes to is, "I'm eating, that's why I'm fat!"

We All Want What We Can't Have

When we label food as "not allowed" we immediately want it more. Suddenly, it's a sacrifice not to have it. The years I spent agonizing over my diet to stay in control, I obsessed about wanting foods I couldn't have. Now that I allow myself to have them, I'm not interested in them. Well, most of them, anyway. The ones I want are truly the ones I want, not the ones I think I want because I can't have them.

Here's an example. When an overeater is exposed to a person who is "policing" the foods they eat, the overeater might only want to eat more. They resist and the result is sad.

A person exposed to a food dictator usually ends up hopelessly obese. They always feel uncomfortable eating so they obsess about food or hide the food they eat so they won't be judged or criticized. Or they just fight back by eating as much as they can in private, sort of a "you can't tell me what to do" nonverbal response.

A more common reaction we may have all experienced is

when someone tells us to stop eating. If I'm having a weak moment when I'm raiding the cookies, my husband might come up to me joking and say, "Put them away, you're going to get fat!" I may have been on my last cookie and already decided I've had enough, but his comment immediately puts me on the defensive. I keep eating just to spite him. How dare he tell me what I can and can't have! (Note to men: Never, ever use the word FAT around your wife, even if you are joking. It is never, ever funny and you will pay for it!)

How Food and Expectations Impact How We Feel About Ourselves

I'm not a psychological expert but I was an emotional eater. I've overcome my emotional issues with food and I have helped others to the same. We don't all have emotional issues with food, but most of us do, at least a little. Maybe you don't even know it.

Emotional baggage can contribute to weight gain. You hear about this in a dramatic sense on talk shows. For example, the 500-pound woman who covers her body in fat because her stepfather raped her when she was 13. No one would dispute the psychological reasons for her obesity, but most of us can't relate because there isn't some profound incident in our lives we could associate with our own weight problem.

Still, little things that happen in our childhood can impact how we view food and ourselves as an adult.

I spoke frankly with a client who told me she always thought she was destined to be a fat adult. When she was a chubby child, her grandmother, although well intentioned, always told her that she was the smart one and that her sister (who was thin) was the pretty one. As a result, she has never felt pretty, even though in reality, most would consider her the prettier one. The negative comments contributed to the negative feelings about herself and sabotaged her ability to achieve her true potential as an adult.

Our personalities are molded as children. Teasing, judging and labeling strongly direct the personality path of the child into adulthood. They believe they are who others say they are. The effects are reversible, but it takes time, education, support and personal evaluation. What doesn't help the situation is another diet.

Valuing Ourselves Through Food

Some of us turn to food for comfort or punishment. We may seek comfort out of boredom or sadness or stress. We may punish ourselves with food because our self-esteem is so low we feel too weak, too worthless, to stop. We sometimes feel being overweight is a brand of shame. We wear it every day and it says, "I'm not a strong person."

It shouldn't be this way. But it is. I was that way. At times, my whole world was about how fat I was getting and the little value I placed on myself for being fat. At other times I was obsessed with the quest for the perfect body as a misguided solution to place more value on myself. It almost defined who I was as a person. Ridiculous, yes, but it's not uncommon.

The funny thing is whether I was fat or thin, I still placed little value on myself. We are disillusioned into believing that the weight is causing our self-esteem problems. Lose the weight and your problems will go away. You will love yourself because you look good.

Is that really all there is? We gain weight so we feel bad about ourselves and eat more and more. We lose weight and we become obsessed, it takes a life of its own and pretty soon you spend six days a week at the gym and stay home on a Saturday night so you don't get tempted to enjoy a piece of pizza or a delicious dessert.

Either way, we use the scale and the mirror to define our self-worth. Whatever happened to just being happy with ourselves? Why don't our talent, our compassion and our kindness define us? Why can't we be happy with our twinkling eyes or our beautiful smile? When did we become so caught up in our bodies? When did we start letting our bodies dictate what kind of person we are?

Comparing Yourself

We are always comparing our bodies to somebody else's. Let's say you are a size 12 and your friend is a size 8. Your friend says, "Ugh, my saddlebags are disgusting!" You immediately think, "If she thinks her thighs are disgusting, what must she think of me?"

While the person might have ulterior motives, most likely the negative comments about herself have nothing to do with the actual size of anyone's thighs but her own. It's mostly about perception of oneself and acceptance. Comments like hers usually stem from her inability to accept herself and her body regardless of reality. It has nothing to do with size or comparison of anyone else.

Contrary to what you may think, a thin person usually doesn't think of themselves as any better than you because of their size. In fact I envied people who could feel good about their bodies even if they were much heavier than me.

Don't take these comments personally. It has nothing to do with you. Defend negative feelings about such comments by thinking about the great qualities in you that aren't defined by something as shallow as a mirror. Don't let these comments get the best of you. Besides, while good health should be a priority, smaller thighs should be at the bottom of the list.

Will Still Another Diet Solve Your Problem?

We try to overcome our negative feelings by trying to lose weight. We assume that if we are thin, our problems will go away. People will like us more, respect us more, love us more.

Anorexics have a problem with their image of themselves. What they see in the mirror is not what others see. Anorexics usually suffer from severe self-esteem issues. They have distorted views of themselves and can't see what's really there. We see a bag of bones; they see a worthless human being. They try to overcome their worthlessness by losing weight. Anorexia has increased because society places a huge value on being thin. Our culture suggests that if they could be thinner they would become a better person.

But that person never exists because the value of oneself only comes from the inside. People with eating disorders need to improve their perception of themselves so they can visually see the person who is really there. *Before anorexics heal by learning how to eat again, they get psychological counseling to figure out why they feel so bad about themselves that they don't eat.*

Overweight people who hate themselves have the same problem; only they eat too much instead of too little. Either way, if they see themselves as a worthless person because of their weight, they will have difficulty being successful at losing weight. If you think you are bad because you eat too much then you have to convince yourself you are a good person as a first step to overcome your problem. There are enough diets and information available to tell us how to do it. We have the solutions; we just aren't empowered to do it.

Did the Diet Do It?

We see testimonials from weight loss winners that say they are happy and love themselves more because they have lost weight. They credit the weight loss plan they used as the reason for their success. But was it the diet? Any diet will work if you stick with it. Are they happy because they lost weight? Or are they happy because they empowered themselves to gain control of their eating problem?

It's like the chicken and egg. Did the success come from the diet or did the success come from finding inner strength to stay with the diet? It's usually both. If you admit that your excessive eating is disabling your happiness and you feel you deserve better, you can establish enough motivation to do something about it. As you feel better about yourself because of the success you have, you are able to gain more control over your eating. Notice I say "feel" better, not "look" better.

Some of us can successfully lose weight but immediately gain it back. We look for the weight loss to make us feel good about ourselves. And when we aren't happy even though we lost weight, we go back to eating more, sometimes more than we did before. Whether you are fat or thin, by dieting, you are looking in the wrong place to find your happiness.

People who are slaves to "diets" usually aren't successful in the long run because they aren't overcoming their food problems; they are just suffering for short periods of time with food deprivation. They may postpone their actions for a while, but usually they go right back to their old habits. The "diet" only perpetuates the obsession. When they fail, they feel worse about themselves.

You need more than a "diet" to cure yourself of the obsession and the negative feelings about yourself. Compulsive overeating damages the quality of life. You have to care enough about yourself and your life to not let food control you. The problem is, it's not something you can just "do."

You can't wake up tomorrow morning and say, "Today I'm going to care about myself" and find joy in something other than food. Even if you have managed to lose weight, you can't fully be liberated unless you rid yourself of the power food has over you.

How Do You Escape the Power of Food?

We all carry different problems and experiences that are the root cause of our food problems. For most of us, the reason isn't profound. It's subtle. You don't have to hate yourself to be a compulsive overeater; if you aren't caring about yourself enough to at least have a generally healthy lifestyle, you need to evaluate why you don't.

Stop thinking your weight is the cause of your problem. If you take the attitude that losing weight will bring happiness, you are fighting a losing battle. Instead of failing at another diet, try to focus on other issues in your life that may contribute to your inability to control the food you eat. If you can feel better about other aspects of your life, you may find the strength to lose weight. Placing little value on yourself and your life can be the medical condition; being overweight is a symptom.

Once you go on medication (i.e., feel worthy or better about yourself), the symptoms subside and you start to feel better. This applies whether you are obese or anorexic. We have a mistaken image of anorexics as starving, ego-minded models. In reality, many are not. Whether you eat too much or eat too little, the underlying problem can be the same. It's about perception of oneself. Food and the mirror are barometers of what kind of person we think we are.

How Do You Know What Your Problem Is?

Start by evaluating yourself, not your weight. Examine your feelings when you know you are going for that binge. Journals are a great way to find your answer. Keep a journal on the kitchen counter and write down the reasons why you are going to eat. I'm not talking about enjoying a treat after dinner. There is a difference between having a few cookies and methodically eating half the bag when you know you've already had enough to eat. And if you are trying hard to lose a few pounds, write down why you consider eating a few cookies is more satisfying to you than getting back in your jeans again. Focus more on yourself, not the food.

Sometimes the problems run deep. If you are a serious

overeater, you may want to seek counseling to help explore your problem.

Using a "Mantra"

A wise person I know achieved weight loss success by repeating a mantra when tempted by food – *will eating get me where I want to be*? Her motivation was not to just lose weight, but to rid herself of the psychological damage and punishment she experienced when she binged. She wanted to lose weight, but more importantly she wanted to overcome the feelings of self-loathing and worthlessness that resulted after binging. Success made her feel better about herself. When she was empowered enough to avoid the binge, she felt positive about herself and eventually succeeded.

One Answer to Two Problems

Eating disorders are quite interesting. I know of someone whose weight and eating problems would swing back and forth. At times she would go for months pigging out every day. At other times she barely ate for months trying to feel in control of life's uncontrollable situations. We can all understand the desire to suppress our emotional pain with chocolate. But it's difficult to understand why someone would become anorexic. Especially when you're talking about someone who can go from one extreme to the other.

She said she felt so good when she didn't eat. "The feeling is euphoric. You feel so in control," she said. The scale became a measurement of her self-worth. She couldn't control the troubling aspects of her life, but at least she was in control of her weight. When she felt weak, she would eat and eat, especially junk food – ***you bad girl!*** When she felt strong she would nearly starve herself – ***you good girl!***

Whether she was anorexic or bingeing, she had issues going well beyond her love of food. No diet in the world was going to help her. We intensely discussed the situation and we both agreed we had a common issue.

When she lost weight, she didn't want to eat normally again because she was afraid of becoming the powerless, chocolate-eating, worthless self that she imagined she was.

When I was obsessed, I feared fattening food or going a day without exercise because I was afraid I would become the chubby, inept child that no one liked again.

We concluded that we both had gone to extremes. We needed to find a "different us." We wanted an "us" that we could love and who could view food in a normal way so we didn't have to be afraid to be "us" anymore.

It's Time to Change Your Thinking

Instead of hating yourself for being overweight, try to feel good about yourself, even if you weigh 300 pounds. Think of the positive things in your life and the good things you have done. If you can't think of anything, then go out and *do something* that makes you feel good about yourself. Don't label yourself as "fat" and "unworthy." Love yourself for all the other good things you are or can be.

If you hate yourself, how are you going to love yourself enough to change? Take a step back, stop focusing on your weight and focus on yourself. Remind yourself that you don't feel the way you do just because you are fat. People think you can't be fat and happy. I think you can. But most of us aren't because being unhappy with ourselves or some aspect of our life is what got us fat in the first place.

If this sounds like you, a diet certainly isn't the answer. The motivation has to be more than "I want to lose weight." You have to want to change how you want to live your life and how you want to feel about yourself. Work on yourself, then work on your weight.

There are hundreds of reasons people have eating problems, but excessive overeating to the point of obesity typically has some psychological origins. We are hiding, hating or feeling "not good enough" or feeling unloved. Food or obesity becomes a shield, a rebellion or a friend. Food provides short-term pleasure and long-term pain.

Getting rid of some of your pain will assist you in getting rid of some of your negative actions. When the pain in you subsides, the power food has over you will also subside. You don't have to be obese to experience this kind of pain. You don't even have to be overweight.

What Have We Learned?

Today's environment has affected how we feel about our relationship with food and ourselves. However, the situation is not uncontrollable. It affects us because we let it affect us. Take some time to analyze your relationship with food. Our expectations, our attitudes about food, our confusion are all changeable.

- Don't define beauty by the media
- You don't have flaws – you have uniqueness
- Learn to live with food
- Don't label foods "good" or "bad"
- Don't let food validate you
- Don't believe a diet will solve your problems
- Figure out your real problems

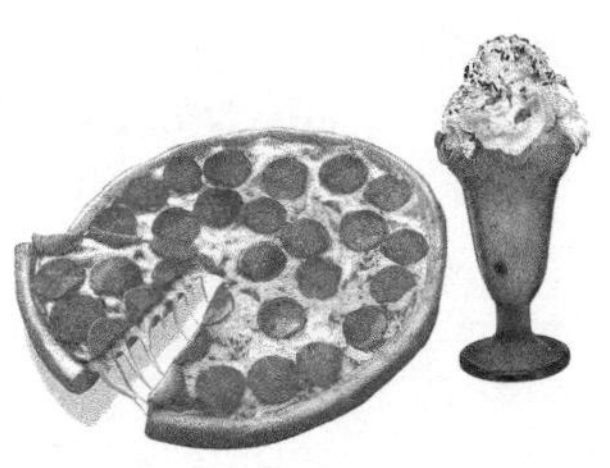

Chapter 9

STEP 2
Identify and Stop
Blame and Denial

When we continuously fail at losing weight, many of us go into denial, or we look for something to blame for our inability to lose weight. We start to blame and deny when we've given up. Usually, the heavier we are, the deeper the denial. If we can conclude there is nothing else we can do about our situation we can give up. "I can't help it because . . . " gives us a reason not to succeed.

I can see why we lie about how much we eat to others, but why do we lie to ourselves? If we could get rid of self-denial and be truthful to ourselves, we'd have a chance for real change. The self-denial factor really sells books and gimmicks. We want to believe it's not what we are eating that is the cause of our weight gain so we look for some other reason we are not losing weight. Blaming allows us to believe our weight problem is caused by a slow metabolism, some missing nutrient or substance in our body or not eating the right combination of foods. We go into denial and don't own up to everything we eat. Many of us could lose weight if we just stopped eating the foods we refuse to admit we eat!

Let's clarify. There is no doubt that some of us are genetically disposed to being heavier. Some people can eat more than others. But if we are in denial we might assume a thin person enjoying a piece of pie can eat whatever they want and it's much more than you! Generally, that's just not true. That's what we want to believe. Even so, while genetics might be an excuse for not being thin, it's not an excuse for being fat and unhealthy.

When we overcome our problem temporarily by losing weight on a diet, we go back into denial when we gain it back. We claim we don't overeat and can't lose weight. Then we lose 20 pounds on a sensible, modified diet like Weight Watchers. The result? We go on and off the Weight Watchers program and never get out of denial and admit that we are eating too much.

We never accept and learn to eat moderately to maintain our weight loss. We go back to our old habits and back to our old "denial" way of thinking. If you are in denial, you can never overcome your problems because you can't admit them.

Sometimes we are not aware that our thoughts or actions are really denial and blame tactics. The actions can be subliminal. Here are a few of the blame and denial tactics I've experienced. Maybe you have too.

Denial

Closet Eating

In the old days I would eat like a bird socially but more than compensate by eating most of my calories when I was alone. This is a common problem for those who are self-conscious about their weight. Maybe we are embarrassed because we fear people will snicker and say, "No wonder she's overweight." Or we might want to communicate to others, "See, my weight problem isn't my fault; look at how little I eat!" Some people will verbally announce to others that they are eating because they "haven't eaten all day!" As if you need an excuse to justify eating!

Comments like these end up drawing more attention to what the person is (or isn't) eating. If they would just keep quiet, no one would even notice how much they are eating. When you are overweight and you "advertise" that you hardly ever eat, people are going to notice.

The worse side of doing this is that when you deprive yourself in public you will typically go out of control when you eat by yourself. The process starts a negative cycle. I ate like this for most of my life. I suffered while passing up a piece of birthday cake at a party only to stop at a bakery and buy a whole one for myself on the way home.

I overcame the problem when I got "out of the closet" and admitted to the world that I do eat. I started to lose weight for me, not for other people. Now I might eat a lot at parties but balance it out when I am alone. I'm not going to skimp on dessert when I'm at a great restaurant and I'm going to sample the hors d'oeuvres my host so generously offered to me at a party.

People say to me, "How can you eat so much and stay thin?" I reply, "Because I watch what I eat at home." I don't want people to assume I can eat whatever I want and not pay for it. Unfortunately, many don't want to believe you because they don't want to admit it to themselves.

If You Don't Use a Plate It Doesn't Count

Food eaten without a plate does not have to be acknowledged. At least that's what most of us think. As long as we eat it over the sink, without a plate, or licked from a spoon it doesn't count.

To this day, I've eaten more ice cream out of the container than in a bowl. I'm still famous for "evening out the cake" too. I've also eaten the equivalent of five Toll House cookies before they even went in the oven. I subconsciously think if I don't actually take a plate the calories don't count.

While I'm still guilty, I've gotten much better about it. The most effective way I stop the action is to first acknowledge what I am doing and then consider if I want to waste my calories unconsciously gobbling them up. Wouldn't I rather sit and enjoy the food I'm eating? If I eat 400 calories of cake an hour before dinner, what's dinner going to taste like? If I can admit to eating it, I can decide whether it's worth eating. If I don't acknowledge what I am eating, I am in denial.

Quantity Denial

Admitting how much of what we eat is probably the most common problem even among people who don't have other denial habits. While nutrition labeling tells us the value of what we are eating, we seem to ignore the serving size on the label. Manufacturers are not dumb. The suggested "serving size" is always limited to a sensible amount of calories but they are unrealistic when considering the average consumption of the product. Who eats a half-cup of ice cream? How about one cookie or a half-cup of cereal?

So for breakfast we think we've eaten a 150-calorie bowl of cereal, when we've actually consumed two, three, maybe even four times that much! I used to measure my cereal, but the serving amount was so little, I'd fudge the measurement but never acknowledge it. It's easy to forget the extra piece, serving or handful of whatever food is most likely one of the causes of our weight problem.

Hiding the Truth Denial

As a personal trainer, I'd ask my clients to keep a food diary for one week to help me identify areas where they could improve their diet. A week later, I'd get a daily food inventory that wouldn't keep a runway model going. It was frustrating. I'd just have to tell them based on what they *said* they were eating, they were already eating a well-balanced diet. Or maybe they weren't eating *enough* calories. Without knowing the facts, I couldn't help them.

I knew they had omitted consciously or subconsciously the extra servings, the fun size candy bars, or the slivers of cake they conveniently forgot or were too embarrassed to admit.

I used to do the same thing. During the years I kept a food journal, I usually admitted to what I ate, but I often didn't account for how much I ate. The more obsessed I got about losing those last 10 pounds, the more in denial I became. The more I tried, the more I denied.

The "But I *Do* Exercise" Denial

We deny how long and how frequently we exercise. We join a gym, say we're going three times a week, but really only go once, then not at all. We buy equipment that collects dust. We show up at an aerobics class once a week, put very little effort into it and stop going because we say it wasn't doing anything. If we own equipment, belong to a gym or are enrolled in an exercise class, we claim we are avid exercisers. We just have been a little too busy lately and will "get back into it" soon. I actually find it refreshing for someone to be honest and say, "My exercise is getting up to change the channel because I'm too lazy to put batteries in the remote." At least they aren't in denial about it.

STEP 2: Identify and Stop Blame and Denial

Most of us say, "I'm not good at exercising." "It's not me." "I'm not like that." You might not be born a natural athlete, but most everyone can exercise. No matter how unathletic you are, you need to exercise to stay healthy and you are able to do it.

"But I *Am* a Healthy Eater" Denial

Do you really eat healthy? How many times a week are you eating broccoli, beans, asparagus, dark green leaf salads, fresh fruit, lean protein and other densely nutritious food? How much calcium are you getting? How much fat are you *really* eating a day? What kind of fat is it? How many times last week did you have pizza, fast food or other fat-laden, nutritiously undesirable food? How many days did you meet the USDA minimum recommended requirements?

So answer the question again. Do you *really* eat healthy? Many of us say we're healthy eaters and do eat healthy some of the time, but many of us are in denial about how much nutritious food we really eat.

There is nothing wrong with eating pizza, chocolate, fat and other fun foods, but the amount and frequency needs to be controlled. We try, but it's just too easy not to eat healthy. So, if we had vegetables with our dinner twice last week and an apple on Tuesday, we claim we are eating healthy. We focus on what we had that was nutritious and forget about how much we ate that wasn't nutritious. Think about it. Does this apply to you?

The Garbage Man

Remember when your mom would say to you, "Finish your plate, there are people starving in Ethiopia!" We were taught to never waste food.

I usually do most of the cooking, shopping and cleaning up after meals. I had a terrible habit of eating small amounts of leftovers after dinner because there was too little to save and I just couldn't throw it out. When it was grocery day and there were only six crackers in the box of Wheat Thins, or a half-serving of Honey Nut Cheerios, I would eat it to get rid of it. If the kids left half a sandwich, I'd eat it instead of throwing it out. I was the garbage disposal!

My actions didn't count as eating food. I was just doing food housekeeping. Those calories didn't count.

I try to remind myself that even if there are starving people, they're not going to get the last glob of mashed potatoes that I'm shoving in my mouth anyway! I toss it in the trash just as easily as I shove it in my mouth. It's gone.

The Blame Game

Similar to denial, blaming takes the responsibility from ourselves by blaming something else for our inabilities to lose weight. "We're fat, but it's not our fault!" We say we are biologically sensitive to carbohydrates; we have bad knees; I don't have time to exercise; I don't have time to cook. We always have an excuse. While sometimes this can be true, often it's not.

Marketing strategies in the diet industry use blame as a way to get you to buy their product. They like to play the blame game with you because you warm up to them. "Poor baby, I understand. Let us help you." They always have a reason why you haven't been successful in the past and it's never your fault. They have discovered the solution for you and it only costs $19.95.

Don't Blame An "Addiction"

The "food addiction" theory allows an overweight person to label their obesity as a disease. It gives them a great excuse to stop trying because when self-labeled, they can stand up and say, "I'm not like you. I'm an addict, it's not my fault!" When they try and fail the "addict" diets, the overeater resigns to being obese. It's a burden that has been placed upon them and they can justify their overeating.

The food addiction theory is unfounded and the unfortunate result is the person usually gets fatter because they have given up. They have an excuse and the diet industry gave it to them.

Don't Blame Your Metabolism

"But it's my metabolism. I can't help it if I'm fat!" We've been using that excuse for years. I remember when I was 10 I used that excuse and I didn't even know what metabolism was.

Lately the medical community is reporting evidence that other biological factors may cause some of us to be fat as well. I'm not challenging the claims, but such theories are providing more excuses for overweight people. If we can blame something, we don't have to do anything about it.

STEP 2: Identify and Stop Blame and Denial

Before you use metabolism, enzymes or genetics as an excuse, ask yourself these questions. Do I exercise regularly? Do I eat a good balanced diet? Do I admit to all the food I eat? Answer these questions, *honestly*. If any, some or all of them are "no," then you can't blame your physiology. If the answer is "yes," then maybe you should consult a medical doctor. Maybe there is a medical reason why you are obese and can't lose weight. Maybe something can be done about it.

Don't Blame Your Aches and Pains

Some people new to exercise stop because they claim they have knee problems or a bad back or some other physical reason. Don't get me wrong, for some of us, it *is* a good reason. But for a lot of us it's a convenient excuse. Most aches and pains we experience after we exercise are because our bodies aren't used to it.

Many of my aerobic students would quit the first week even though they loved the program. Typically, they tried to do too much too soon. Their muscles got a little sore and so they quit. Some were fearful that the discomfort would lead to injury. In most cases, the reality is they are experiencing discomfort only because the muscles are weak and not used to the activity. With exercise and strength training, the body would become more resistant to injury. If they started at a lower intensity and learned how to perform the movements correctly, they could strengthen the muscles and reduce the chance of real problems.

Some people really do have medical issues, but don't let the initial soreness become an excuse for giving up.

Don't Justify Your Actions

We often try to justify our actions. We justify why we are eating, what we are eating and how much we are eating. We're at a party, out to dinner with friends, having pizza on Friday night and we justify overeating by saying we can't diet right now. "I'll diet tomorrow," we promise. But tomorrow never comes. We always have an excuse for why we are overeating.

I used to eat one fourth of a cake because I wanted to get rid of it. The cake was tempting me so I figured I'd just eat it now and then I could get back on my diet. I justified eating 900 calories now so I wouldn't eat 900 calories later. How bizarre is that!

The Pizza and Ice Cream Diet

We justify super sizing to save a buck. We eat two Egg McMuffins because it was two for $2.00 and we couldn't pass up the deal. We justify eating junk foods because they are convenient and quick. We argue that nutritious food is less convenient and more expensive. But consider how much money you spend on junk and high priced take-out dinners. Think of how much money you spend on other unnecessary items in your life. If healthier food does cost more, aren't you and your family worth it?

Don't Plan Then Blame

We are busy so we plan everything and make it so complicated we can't possibly execute the plan. Then we blame our failure on our busy lives or our hectic lifestyle that got in the way of our plan.

With exercise, we want to lose weight quickly so we figure the more we exercise the faster we will get results. With dieting, we map out a strategy, follow an unrealistic low-calorie diet and then decide when we're going to do it. "I'll start my diet on Monday" and then eat everything in sight like it's Fat Tuesday.

The mindset leads to the thinking that it will be over some day.

We think we have to plan to lose weight. We join a gym, go four times the first week, are sore as hell, and a month later we're not going at all. Then we spend a year saying, "Yeah, I've got to get back into it." We feel we have to have some sort of self-made contract signed in order to get off our butt!

Gyms and aerobic classes are packed on January 2 carrying out everyone's New Year's Resolutions and by mid-February, only a few remain. Everyone goes back in May with hopes of losing weight for bathing suit season, and when they don't get the results they want (remember they want to do it in a month) they give up, buy a bigger suit and stop going. Then of course, you've got the kids all summer, no time for yourself. Then we go back in September once the kids are in school and by the end of October after we've eaten all the kids' Halloween candy we say, "I'll get back into it after Christmas" and the cycle starts again.

We set ourselves up for failure. We make it all so complicated. There's nothing wrong with joining a gym, but if you don't have time to take a walk, how are you going to have time to drive to a gym? If you're planning to go on a diet but postpone it this week because you have two birthday parties, a lunch with a friend and three soccer games with drive-thru dinners, how do you expect to succeed?

Don't Blame the Restaurants

We eat out often and we rely on restaurants to nourish us. Blaming our frequent restaurant visits for our tightening belts is a common excuse.

It is harder to control your caloric intake when healthier, lower calorie alternatives are limited – sometimes nonexistent. While restaurants should be conscientious about the nutritional quality of the food they serve, I think we are mostly to blame. We blame restaurants for not offering healthy alternatives, but the reality is there is little demand for healthy food. Look around. What sells? Fat and sugar! When fast food chains try to experiment with healthier alternatives they're pulled six months later for lack of sales.

I recently read about a restaurant that offered a few "heart healthy" dishes for customers. Sales of the entree were flat but the chef still felt they were very good-tasting dishes. He offered the same entree without labeling them "healthy." Guess what? Sales for the dishes rose dramatically!

We want quantity. We control how much we eat and we want as much as we can get on a plate and a side as well. Food is always available. It's up to us to control how much actually goes in our mouth.

The food industry is there to make money. If we didn't buy it, they wouldn't sell it.

Are You Willing to Be Honest?

Does any of this apply to you? Are you blaming and denying? Are you being truthful with yourself? Being dishonest with yourself is self-destructive and a waste of time. Who are you kidding? Does it really matter to anyone but you?

Stop the blaming and denying. It's the moment of truth. If you can't admit you are eating too much and you don't believe you can control your situation you will never overcome your problem.

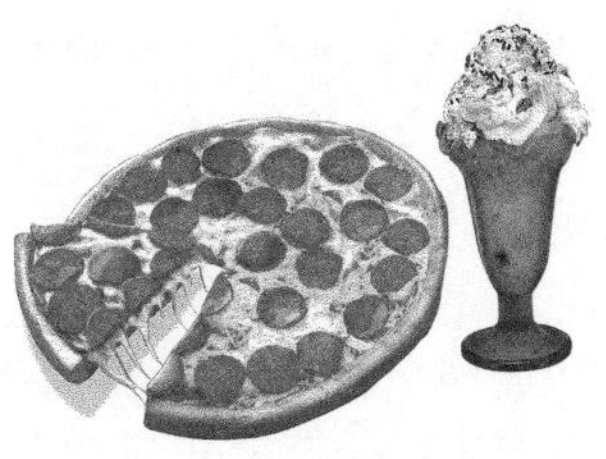

Chapter 10

STEP 3
Accept Realities and Move On

To start making changes in your life, *real changes*, you have to face reality. You need to recognize the limitations that exist in our effort to reach our goals. You need to accept and identify:

- What you can achieve
- What makes you achieve success
- How quickly you can make changes
- How you measure success

If you can understand and accept these realities, you will find it easier to meet your goals.

What You Can Achieve

Unrealistic Expectations

Our expected goals have become unrealistic. For many of us our expectations are not only hard to achieve but impossible.

The reality is hard to accept when that's not the message we are getting from the media and society – and especially the diet industry. We believed their exaggerated "guaranteed" claims and when we didn't meet our expectations we blamed ourselves or made excuses for our failures. In the process, achieving the goal of a healthy body fell by the way side and we stopped trying.

While our genetic history doesn't make us unhealthy and fat, it does dictate how easily we put on weight, our body fat levels and our overall shape.

We Come In All Sizes and Shapes

Some of us are pear shaped with wider hips and legs; some are apple shaped with thin legs and a wider middle. Some of us are large chested; some of us are flat chested. You get my point. Yes, with a lot of work you can reshape your body to a degree. But no matter how dedicated you are, your genetics will only let you go so far.

Body fat levels are genetic. Some people are able to put on lean muscle easier than others. Some people have an athletic figure and seem to be able to get definition in their arms with three months of moderate weight lifting and little change in diet. Others spend years in the gym and follow a strict diet but still don't achieve the same results.

The Endless Search for Perfection

Accepting this reality, disappointing as it was, helped me come to terms with my imperfect body. After a lifetime of feeling fat, I wanted to find out how it felt to be, not only average weight, but to overcome my genetic obstacles and pursue aesthetic perfection. The diet industry told me it could be done. In my 30's already, time was running out. I was mentally ready to take on any challenge in pursuit of an awesome body. (It's still hard to believe I was so compelled to accomplish such a meaningless goal.) With a lot of hard work and sacrifice I overcame my genetic obstacles to a certain degree but I never achieved the body I really wanted.

I thought the inability to achieve my goals was my fault. After all, I really didn't have the *perfect* diet. I ate way too many desserts at Grandma's house and I'd have a binge here and there. I'd think, "If you had only been more disciplined, you could have done it." I viewed my imperfection or inability to achieve my goals as a weakness in me. It didn't matter that everyone around me either admired me for my accomplishments or didn't take notice and wouldn't care to begin with.

Would it have been possible for me to achieve the body I wanted? I'll never know. I really don't care anymore. I do know that in order to get the body I fantasized about I would have to do more than lift weights, exercise a lot and eat a strict diet. With a healthy weight and a lot of lean mass, I still have beefy thighs and a lot of cellulite. In order for me to lose the excess weight in my thighs, I would have to lose a lot of weight – more than I should. Even if I were stranded on a deserted island for 6 months eating nothing but bugs and berries, you'd still see fat bulges on my thighs!

Paying a High Price

But is it worth it? The price I would have to pay is to stop enjoying food. I would have to be intensely aerobic and dedicated for the rest of my life. At that point, it's not about having a very healthy lifestyle; it's about forcing your body to do something it doesn't want to do. It's very liberating to let go of the goal. Even if I had reached the goal I would obsess about losing it. And besides, the only person that cares is me. So if I can be happy and accept my imperfect body then everyone else will too.

Don't get me wrong, there is nothing wrong with a person who enjoys heavy physical exercise and maintaining a rigid diet as long as they have a healthy view of themselves. *Why* they are doing it is the subtle, but *major* difference.

It's frustrating but the reality is that some of us have to work harder than others and sometimes we just have to accept who we are and love ourselves for who we are. Life is too short to worry about something you can't change. If you are eating right and getting regular exercise, you should be proud at what you have accomplished and be happy with the best you can be. So if your best is a size 14, then you should try to be a healthy size 14 and feel good about it.

Set Points Do Exist

I am convinced we all have weight set points that are difficult to move or reset. You can do it, but most likely your body will continue to resist it.

Refusing to accept my set point contributed to my obsession and my feelings of inadequacy and failure. The diet industry made me believe that set points didn't exist. I could get the body I always wanted, if only I used their equipment, took their pill or followed their diet. I now accept my set point and I am happy with it.

I consider my set point to be between 145-150. If I eat moderately and exercise regularly, my average weight is 145. If I overeat my weight goes up a bit. When I eat less or excessively exercise for a period of time, my weight goes down, but it goes back up as soon as I resume my regular eating habits.

When I was unhappy with my weight at 145, I tried to get down to 140. For several years I tried to decrease my weight only 5 pounds. I tried everything I could and even when I was on *Body for Life* (the most serious I had ever been), I never reached the goal. I did lose a little, but at what price?

I lived for my body. I was held captive by the quest. I had developed an unhealthy power struggle with food. I lifted and exercised to exhaustion. And with all this, I still didn't feel good about myself.

It's been over two years since I stopped trying to change my set point. I enjoy all food, I exercise moderately and I take no supplements other than a daily vitamin and calcium. I haven't gained a pound.

I no longer obsess to squeeze into a size 6. I'm happy wearing a size 8 because it is more comfortable. Most importantly, I am a much happier person and have a healthier relationship with food.

What Is Your Set Point?

But is your set point really your set point? You really won't know until you *honestly* evaluate your current lifestyle. If you consistently eat a healthy, moderate calorie diet and exercise regularly, then the weight you maintain is most likely your set point.

So, if you've honestly tried everything to get rid of those last few pounds unsuccessfully, you might just want to accept that your body was meant to be that way. Maintain your set point; eat healthy and exercise ***for your health*** and get on with your life.

A Beautiful Example

A good example of larger, healthy beauty is the model Emme. She's the Saudi Arabian-born, plus-sized model who hosts (or did host) a makeover fashion program on the E! Entertainment channel. I wish she and other larger role models would get more positive publicity. Emme looks fantastic at a size 14 (thereabouts). She is an average sized normal woman most of us can relate to. She's absolutely radiant! She looks happy, healthy and sexy – like she'd really be fun to be with. She's probably happier than most models because she can eat!

But even though Emme is not a size 6 she still takes care of herself. People clearly see the difference even if it's not in her dress size. Emme is a healthy woman who doesn't have a slim build. She doesn't spend her time with unnecessary sacrifices in pursuit of an unrealistic expectation. She is positive about her larger self so the media leaves her alone. It's not worth saying anything negative about her weight, because they know she is comfortable with it. I would love to see her with an exercise and nutrition video instead of Cindy Crawford!

Just because you can't be thin doesn't mean you can't be beautiful and just as happy. But, you still need to eat a balanced diet and exercise. It's one thing to be a healthy size 14; it's another to be a lethargic, fast food eating size 14. You can see the difference. Not only that, but the latter will eventually be a size 22 unless a lifestyle change is made.

Reveal Your Inner Beauty

Be realistic and strive to be a healthier, more energetic person. It has no down side. Your self-esteem will be better; you will be happier and have more fun. Don't dictate your self-worth by a number on a scale or a dress size like I did for most of my life. Because I was a chubby child with low self-esteem, I couldn't see the positive, energetic person I had become. I focused on my flaws as a weakness in me instead of a genetic reality. I obsessed and beat myself up trying to achieve the unachievable. When I gave up the obsession and started to accept my flaws as an unchangeable reality, I started to see a better me. And others saw a better me even though I was the same size.

The bottom line is that if you free yourself of unrealistic expectations, you can focus on the obtainable. But if the realistic obtainable doesn't make you happy, then you need to travel inward to discover why you can't be happy with the body God has given you.

What Makes You Achieve Success

What actually causes us to lose weight? We've been avoiding the truth by believing remedies that don't exist. It's time we get back to reality and review how we actually lose weight.

Calories In; Calories Out

There are two components to losing weight: calories in, calories out. To lose a pound you have to eat 3,500 fewer calories or expend 3,500 more calories. You can't burn more calories by popping a pill or eating a special combination of foods. The only way you can lose weight is to either reduce caloric intake or increase caloric expenditure. In other words, you need to eat fewer calories and/or exercise.

Accepting the Reality of the Calorie

Somewhere down the line, "calorie" became a dirty word. People hate counting calories so every successful diet plan hides the reality of the calorie. It's time we accept the calorie again. Avoiding the "calorie" is avoiding the issue.

The calorie is used as a measurement for all foods: nine calories per gram of fat, four calories per gram of carbohydrates, four calories per gram of protein and seven calories for a gram of alcohol. If you limit carbohydrates you limit calories; if you limit fats, you limit calories; if you limit protein, you limit calories; and if you limit alcohol, you limit calories. So instead of eliminating foods from your diet, foods that you may enjoy, why don't you just eat what you want and keep your total calories in check?

Good Food Doesn't Equal "0" Calories

Many of us have the perception that "healthy" foods are low in calories and we can eat as much as we want. I have to be careful how I say this: sometimes that's not true. I've watched persistent, yet nonsuccessful dieters eat a huge fruit salad for lunch and then, unsatisfied, eat handfuls of Doritos. They may admit to the Doritos, but they don't consider the fruit salad calories. Fruit is fairly caloric and if eaten in large quantities, the calories add up. An apple, pear, orange or banana contains about 80-100 calories. If you eat five fruits per day, that's almost 500 calories.

I'm not saying you shouldn't eat five servings of fruit, but you do have to account for it. And while fruit is a satisfying ender to a lunch, for most of us only fruit for lunch is unfulfilling – resulting in the Doritos slip. A turkey sandwich would have been a more satisfying choice and you'd still be able to have a little fruit along with it and consume fewer calories in the long run.

Reading It Wrong

The low-fat craze got everyone to read labels. As long as the food was low fat nothing else mattered. We started to ignore the calories in the food because calories became irrelevant. Now we know better. The difference between a fat-free cookie and a regular cookie is usually only about 10-20 calories per serving. There may be a significant reduction in the fat amount, but low-fat foods often have higher sugar content so the net calorie difference is pretty insignificant. So you're giving up a better tasting cookie to save a few calories. And most of us end up eating more cookies because of our misleading perception that a low-fat cookie is better for us. Not to mention you're not getting the taste satisfaction of a really good cookie.

If you look at a nutritional label, every food component listed can be transformed into a calorie. All food components listed are in grams. Learn how to read a nutrition label. You'll discover that no matter how you disguise it, the calorie is what counts.

Exercise – The Other Dirty Word

For most of us, our bodies need 1,200 calories a day just to support our BMR (Basal Metabolic Rate). BMR is the amount of energy your body requires every day to perform its most basic functions, i.e., breathing, digesting, circulation, etc., without any physical activity. Physical movement is required in order to add more calories to your body's daily needs without gaining weight. Therefore, the more you move, the more calories your body needs (i.e., the more you can eat!).

An average woman should be able to consume about 1,800 - 2,000 calories a day and maintain her weight. However, because so many of us are barely moving each day, our bodies don't need that many calories. In fact some of us move so little, we don't need much more than what our bodies need to function.

Accept the reality that unless you want to eat like a bird for the rest of your life, you are going to have to move your body more.

How Quickly We Can Change It

Realistic Expectations for Results

Based on marketing hype for various diets and products, we have impossible expectations of how quickly we can lose weight.

The typical message is that success is easy and it can be obtained in 30 days. So we set out to accomplish our weight loss goal by drastically changing our diet overnight and suffer in hopes of obtaining fast goals that are impossible to meet.

You need to set your goals to reflect how much effort you are willing to put in to reach it. If you are a size 16 and believe you can be a size 6 in three months you need to recognize that the reality is it's going to take a lot of work to accomplish your goal – much more than you think. You won't achieve such an aggressive goal just by walking 30 minutes on a treadmill three times a week and adhering to a low-calorie diet; well most of the time, except for the birthday celebration on Tuesday and the dinner with appetizers and dessert on Saturday and don't forget the pizza and the popcorn at the movie on Friday.

If you can ignore the hype and look at the math, you will begin to recognize the truth. It takes 3,500 fewer calories to lose a pound. An average day's calories are about 1,800-2,500. Theoretically, if your average caloric intake today is 2,500 calories per day (that's a lot), you couldn't lose 30 pounds if you didn't eat a speck of food for a month!

Of course that's dramatic, but do you see what I mean? What the heck do we expect? Think how long it took you to gain that weight. Add to it the fact it's a lot easier to eat 500 more calories per day than eat 500 fewer calories per day. If you religiously ate 500 fewer calories per day and expended 500 calories more a day, you could lose 2 pounds a week. That's about 8 pounds a month. Using this example losing 30 pounds would take you about four months.

While the above figure is theoretically achievable, the chance of avoiding backslides during that long grind is unrealistic. Think about it. Is it realistic to assume you are going to eat 500 fewer calories and expend 500 more calories *every* day for four months?

It doesn't matter if you are trying to lose 5 or 500 pounds; the mechanics of losing weight are the same. However, the time it takes to lose weight differs depending on your current caloric intake. It sounds so incredible when you hear about a person who lost 75 pounds in six months, but if you look at the math it makes sense. Most diets try to keep you in a caloric range of 1,200-1,500 calories a day. If you're 75 pounds overweight you are most likely eating a lot of calories a day.

STEP 3: Accept Realities and Move On

Let's say you currently eat about 3,500 calories a day. You could lose about 3 pounds a week and still be eating 2,000 calories a day. But, if you are trying to lose 10 pounds, average 1,800 calories a day and cut back 500 calories to 1,300 per day, it's going to take you almost three months just to lose the 10 pounds.

But it's hard to cut your diet back to just 1,300 calories a day. If you cut back much more, you risk sending your body into a "starvation" mode that will slow down your metabolism. Not to mention you'll be pretty darn hungry. Losing any more weight almost has to be an exact science with no margin for error (i.e., no cheating). That's why it's so hard to lose those last 5 or 10 pounds we *think* we need to lose. And remember, one day of "going off your diet" has to be factored into the equation.

One Bad Day Can Ruin the Whole Week

Going "off" of your diet can be as subtle as a few hundred calories in extra cookies one day to eating an extra 2,000 calories. Looking at the math again, let's assume you have been good all week and, after a little cheating here and there, your net reduction in calories averages about 300 calories a day. On Sunday, you give yourself a day off and go hog wild at an all you can eat brunch buffet. You have eggs benedict, home fries, a couple sausages, a waffle with blueberries and whipped cream, and sample four or five desserts (sounds like a lot but in the past give me the green light and I could easily put that much away).

There is nothing wrong with having a grand splurge now and then but just remember that one excessive meal can ruin an entire week of being "good."

Reality Bites

So what's realistic? The grim reality is a weight loss of about 1 or 2 pounds a week is about the best you can do, depending on your eating and exercise habits. Most likely, it will take much longer.

If you try to dramatically reduce your food intake or deprive yourself of foods you enjoy, losing 30 pounds will be grueling and unrealistic. The problem with doing this is that you find it is just too hard to diet. Then you either give up or go into a starve/binge mode causing you to be a habitual dieter. You start feeling like the word "diet" is synonymous with "die-*ing*." Changing your weight shouldn't be a punishment. You can only punish yourself for so long. Changing to a healthier lifestyle might take longer, but at least you can enjoy the ride.

The Key Is to Start with Baby Steps

You can't run a marathon if you can't run around the block. A big problem with our goal setting is that we set out to accomplish too much. Going from a fried food, emotional eater to a poached salmon, power walking eater overnight is unrealistic. By thinking you can change overnight, you are setting yourself up for failure.

Let's say you have your "wake up call." You say, "This is it. I can do this! Starting tomorrow, I'm going to lose 20 pounds!" You're spiritually changed, throw out all your junk food and plan to start a new life. But within a week you're back to your old habits. You make a commitment to change and two days later you have a weak moment where you raided the cookie jar. Then at your next meal you find yourself finishing off the last of the bloomin' onion with a smile on your face and a sadness in your heart. Failed again. You only feel worse than you did before and your confidence dwindles with every failed attempt.

While you can make a decision to change, for the most part, you can't just say it and change it. Being successful is about failing, succeeding and failing again, but never giving up. If you need to lose 30 pounds, you've got to learn how to do it, have the stamina to do it and care about it enough to stick with it. You have to think positively and believe you can do it. Never give up.

You may say, but I *do* keep trying. I am always trying to lose weight. I start a diet and then within a few days, I'm off of it and pigging out again.

I compare it to my kids and sports. They want to play soccer but when they aren't as good as everyone else they want to quit. They want to be the best soccer player but they don't want to put the time in or learn how to play the game. They want it to be easy.

Quitting Before You Start

When you expect yourself to suddenly be good at losing weight, you set yourself up for disappointment. We look for some miraculous power in us to be successful and lose weight and, for most of us, it doesn't happen. And when it doesn't happen we quit. We may start over, but we never learn anything in the process. We just keep quitting because we failed instead of learning from our failures how to be successful.

If you are used to eating a donut for breakfast, a hero sandwich and chips for lunch, a Snickers bar at mid-afternoon and can't seem to end the day without a half a dozen cookies, then how are you supposed to eat egg whites, salad and an apple instead? You've got to have some serious motivation behind you to accomplish that. Even if you are good for a couple of days, your cravings, habits and hunger will take over and you will dig into those cookies or swing through the drive-thru window and have a relief-seeking binge.

Gradual Changes Work

We want to change our junk food, couch potato habits, and we want to do it *today*. That's a big demand you place on yourself. You want to eat healthier so you throw out the cookies, chips and fried food and expect to overhaul your diet overnight. You can't eat any of your favorite foods so you weaken and give in to temptation before nightfall.

Instead, take small steps in the right direction. Don't super size your lunch today and have one less cookie; prepare a fresh vegetable every night or always order a side of vegetables at a restaurant; pull some cheese off of your sandwich or cut back on the mayonnaise. If you feel depressed and are wallowing in a tub of ice cream stop yourself at two servings before you add to the damage by eating more. And then be proud of yourself for doing it.

The same principle applies to an exercise program. Joining a gym requires a large time and financial commitment. Many who join end up not going at all. If you've ever used the excuse that you are too busy and then join a gym as an answer to your problems, you are pursuing the wrong solution. You've just added up to an hour to your busy schedule just getting back and forth to the gym. I'm not saying don't join a gym, but if time is a problem, why don't you start with a set of dumbbells. Learn to use them by watching an ESPN weight program and start walking around the block. Why don't you just do something more than you were before and be proud of yourself for doing it!

By taking baby steps, you slowly learn how to control your food day-by-day, week-by-week. Find joy in the short walk you took and try to go a little further the next time. If you get distracted and don't walk for three days, don't get down on yourself and quit – walk again on the fourth day. Instead of focusing on the mental "sacrifice" of choosing healthier options, focus on how much better you feel after making that choice.

When you pig out, try to pig out a little less than you did before. And if you don't, accept it as a setback, but keep going. Start small and never give up.

How We Measure Success

Success should be measured by the change in the quality of your life, not by a number on the scale. Better health, improved energy and a more positive attitude is long-lasting success. Changing your weight by a diet gives you a false sense of security. It's only temporary. Chances are your success will turn to failure again.

Don't Measure Success by the Scale

Measuring and weighing yourself and basing success on the two can do more harm than good. We obsess about seeing results by something tangible like a scale or tape measure instead of how we feel.

My obsession got to the point that the scale or tape measure was the indicator of what my day was going to be like. If I weighed 144, I was happy, had energy and bounced and smiled through the day. If I was 149 I was sluggish, felt hopeless and thought I was a bad, weak person – even if I knew the weight gain was a result of temporary water retention.

When I was on *Body for Life* and had a set goal, I tortured myself numerous times a day waiting for that magic number (the goal) to appear on the bathroom scale. It never did.

The goal consumed me. As time began to run out, I grew frantic. Right before the end of my three-month "transformation" period, I took laxatives and water pills in hopes of seeing the magic number on the scale.

I found the tape measure to be similar. I could measure my waist one day and it would be 27 inches. The next day it would read 27.5 inches due to water gain, what I had for dinner, pre-period, whatever. It's also very easy to fudge a measuring tape as it can fluctuate, like our weight, several times a day. But, unlike the scale, I could manipulate the measurement based on how I wanted to feel about myself that day.

I would use the measuring tape as a barometer of my self-worth – whether I was a "good girl" or a "bad girl." If I wanted to feel good about myself, I could stand straight and hold my stomach in and measure a 27-inch waist. If I wanted to beat myself up, I could slouch and release the muscles, and the tape could read as high as 29.5 inches.

As a personal trainer I was tempted to fudge my clients' results just to make them feel better about themselves. It would probably have been in their best interest and they would have been none the wiser.

I'm not concluding that we should never weigh or measure ourselves. It's just that when we rely on the scale to dictate our progress, we can become discouraged and give up. If you are on a diet, the scale matters because you are waiting to reach a number so you can go off the diet. The mirror and the scale don't mean anything if you don't like the changes in your behavior.

When you change your lifestyle, the scale becomes secondary. The success in feeling better and taking care of your body comes first. The scale will cooperate if you continue to make positive changes. But since you aren't dieting, the changes may take longer. It takes longer, but if you make the changes gradually and don't sacrifice, the journey is a good one – one that you won't ever want to end. If you are dieting, the journey is full of sacrifice, punishment and distress and you can't wait for it to be over. Which road do you want to take?

What Have We Learned?

- You can only achieve *your* potential not someone else's
- It's going to take time to change so it's important to like the changes. Enjoy the ride
- You can't change your lifestyle overnight. Make gradual changes and adapt to your new lifestyle
- Change will not happen unless you apply the principles of losing weight
- Measure success by your changed life, not by the changes in the mirror

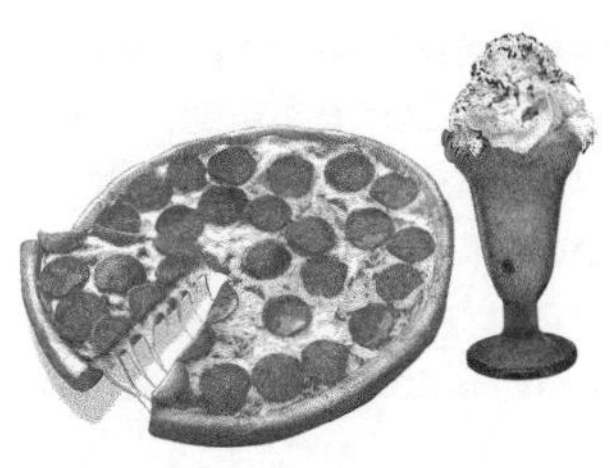

Chapter 11

STEP 4
Getting Ready for Change

Lifestyle change has a beginning, but it has no end. You don't stop and start again. You don't get back into it. You don't give up. You live it. Every day.

Does lifestyle change mean you have to eat only healthy foods, stick to a precise exercise program and be good all the time? No it doesn't. It's changing how you view yourself and food by implementing and adapting to changes in your lifestyle, making you a healthier person.

It's learning how to find moderation in a country where there is always a more convenient way to eat and to move. Our environment does not have to dictate how we live. Today's environment can be destructive and it's up to each individual to find a balance between our wants and needs.

A big part of changing to a healthier lifestyle is improving your eating habits and moving your body more. It's taking care of yourself. The problem is we really don't want to change. We say we want to change, but we don't want to give up the lifestyle we are accustomed to. We think living a healthier lifestyle is a sacrifice. We believe we aren't a "healthy living" kind of person and we aren't capable of change.

Up until now, the process has been to change the way you think and feel about your situation and yourself. It helped you to recognize how our environment has caused us to be obsessed, resistant, confused and hopeless to change. It explained the mental reaction of denial and blame as an excuse for giving up. And put you back in reality by showing realistic expectations in achieving your own potential so you can move forward with a new honest, realistic approach to your situation.

So now that you understand why you feel the way you do, you have to convince yourself you are capable of change. You have to get mentally prepared to change.

Preparing for Change

This step is the most important path to success. By mastering this step you will be able to cross over to The NEW You. It's not about wanting to lose weight, but wanting to change your life. While it can be the hardest step, if you are able to succeed, the actual doing is easy. You have to be mentally ready to make the changes that will impact your life. You need to realize that you *can* do it and you *want* to do it.

Start by answering the following questions. Analyze your current thinking about your answers and then try to change your answers.

- Why don't you want to change?
- Is your lifestyle keeping you from change?
- What's not to like?

Why Don't You Want to Change?

I can't do it. It's too hard. I don't have time. I'm a food addict. My body is resistant to exercise. I'm not that kind of person. If the answer to the question sounds like one, some or all of these, you can change but you are using an excuse not to change.

But what if you eliminate the excuses and change the answer? I can do it. It's not that hard. I do have the time. I'm not a food addict. My body does want to exercise. I *am* that kind of person. If you can change your attitude, you can change your answer.

Is Your Lifestyle Keeping You from Change?

We talked about how our external environment keeps us from change but what about your own personal environment? How are you living your personal life? What kind of person do you think you are? What kinds of things or people make you happy and are they in your life? Do you have any dreams? Can you rekindle those dreams? Can you find new ones?

Do you feel incapable of change? Are you feeling hopeless? Is your lifestyle feeding those feelings? If you reconsider what kind of person you are or wish to be and take action in changing your own personal environment (how you think, feel and live day to day) it will help you believe you can change.

In order to change, your surroundings have to change. The environmental influences will always be there (Hollywood, McDonald's, the diet theory of the week). You have to change your own personal environment – move it towards a healthier place. Look around you. Where do you find joy – where do you find sadness? Put yourself in a better position to achieve change.

What's Not to Like?

Common answers to this question: I won't like the change. I don't want to give up eating everything I want. It would be a sacrifice.

While you may think you don't want to, ask yourself, "Do I like the way I feel now? Am I really happy living like this?"

I played golf with a guy (a stranger) one day – I was walking, he was driving a cart. He offered to share his cart with me, but I said, "No, I like to walk." He said, "Yeah, I used to walk a few years ago. I used to walk three miles every morning." "Why did you stop?" I asked. "Well, I got sidetracked for a few weeks and I just haven't got back into it." "How did you feel when you were walking?" I questioned. "I felt great. It was wonderful! I was in much better shape, I had more energy." "So if it felt so good, why aren't you doing it now?" I goaded. "Oh, I'll get back into it someday," he said. "Why not tomorrow?" I asked. "Yeah, maybe," he replied with a bit of embarrassment.

Do you hear how silly this sounds? Why would he *not* want to do something that made him feel good? Why do we prefer to live a life that is not as enjoyable as the life we could live?

Eating is the same. Isn't it better to leave the table feeling satisfied rather than spending the next several hours feeling stuffed and sluggish? Isn't it better to not have regrets?

The Path Forward

There is a path that leads to a healthier life and it doesn't have to involve running three miles every day or giving up pizza and ice cream. The strategy in getting you ready for change is to rethink your answers to the preceding questions. The following will help lead you in that direction.

- Stop dieting
- Make a decision
- Redefine yourself and understand you can change
- Redefine your life
- Be prepared for setbacks

Stop Dieting

The term "going on a diet" implies you are doing something short term you don't want to do. Going "on a diet" means you expect to go "off the diet." If your goal is to finish the diet, most likely you will fail.

Changing the way we eat and move are part of the change, but not the only priority. Losing weight occurs when you decide to change other aspects of your life. "Diets" produce the thinking that you'd be happy if only you could lose weight. The truer part of losing weight has more to do with the improved way of life, not the thinner image in the mirror. You can't be a thin person unless you live like a thin person.

Did you ever notice a lot of diet commercials' "after" pictures show not only a thinner person, but also an athletic one? They'll show the "transformed" person hiking up a hill, jogging, enjoying a salad on the tennis court. They'll talk about the energetic life they lead now that they are thin. It makes one believe that going on a diet changes your life. Going on a diet doesn't make you change. Only *you* make yourself change.

There has to be more to the equation than denying yourself food. You have to be able to live with the change. You have to incorporate eating and activity changes as part of your daily life – a *joyous* part of your life. Focusing too much on "losing weight" actually causes us to gain weight and is contributing to the obesity problem in this country. It's best to remove your focus from food or how intensely you need to exercise. We start thinking about it too much and we only want food more because we can't have it. We resist exercising because we *have* to do it.

Make a Decision

What are you going to do to change? Be honest with yourself.

STEP 4: Getting Ready for Change

Change is only going to happen if you make it happen. If you need to lose 30 pounds and you know you aren't willing to give up your current lifestyle *forever*, then accept it's not going to happen. Forget dieting. You are better off not even trying because the inevitable failure will only make you feel worse about yourself and you will likely become more obsessed with food.

If you need to lose 30 pounds and you tell yourself you can't do it, then you won't. If you are always willing to find your next excuse, then you will always use that excuse for your failure. You've got your decision and your excuse all ready; it's just a matter of timing. At what point are you going to use your "excuse" playing card?

Before you start the lifestyle change process, make a firm decision that you *can* do it. I don't mean setting a goal. I mean mentally preparing yourself to live differently. Accept that you will live differently and there is no going back. Food will always be there. The couch is always an option. You have to convince yourself that you want to live a different way. You need to embrace the positive side of change, never the negative. Actually, there is no negative side other than the incorrect messages you mentally give yourself.

Lifestyle change doesn't just involve changing how you eat and how you move. You have to change how you view yourself and decide how you want to live. You need to change how you think in order to set the stage for change.

Be Accountable Only to Yourself

Make the decision to change and make it only for yourself. Many of us want to tell everyone we are on a diet. In most cases, it's the kiss of death. Keep it to yourself. This is for you. It's personal. If you tell everyone you are on a diet you immediately put pressure on yourself.

Have you ever told people you were on a diet and a month later feel foolish when you haven't lost weight (or gained back weight you lost) and then be embarrassed to eat in front of them? Now you must not only admit your failure to yourself, but you have to tell the world. You mentally start dieting for other people, not for you. You start playing the role in front of others and then childishly cheat on yourself when you are alone.

If you keep it to yourself and you are successful, people will notice. Bask in your glory after you've succeeded.

Change "I Have To" Into "I Want To"

Wanting to do something is easier than *having* to do something. Most people who want to lose weight start their day by saying, "I have to start another diet today," or, "I have to exercise today." You are immediately setting yourself up for failure because you've already defined it as something you don't want to do. Focus on what you can have, not what you can't have. Look forward to having a good healthy dinner after a pleasant walk with your neighbor.

If you don't want to change because you think you prefer your life as it is, answer this question honestly: Do you ever wish you were more energetic, that you were capable of controlling your food and would naturally want to live a healthier life? If the answer is yes, then you do care about how you are living your life. You are resisting because you consider changing your lifestyle as something you *have* to do. If you don't believe you will like the change, then why *would* you want to change? But if you *want* to change your behaviors, you can and I *guarantee* you will like it.

Redefine Yourself and Understand You Can Change

Getting the upper hand on your weight also means you'll have to take control of how you *define* yourself. Lots of weight losing wannabes start their program in a hopeless abyss of poor self-esteem. "I don't believe I can do it." "It's too hard." "I'm not an exercise person." "I'm too old, too fat, too out of shape." They can't imagine themselves a healthy, active person. That's someone else.

So the first thing you need to do is understand that you *can be* a healthy, active person. Forget about the goal of losing weight. For now, start acting like a healthy, active and happier person.

No matter how large you are, do not accept that you are hopelessly fat. If you act fat, you can't act thin. Do not self-chastise by speaking negatively about your body or your physical abilities. Do not compare yourself to anyone else. Do not put yourself down. Feed your starving ego only the most positive of messages.

It's hard to believe now that one day you could actually want to go to the gym or choose the grilled chicken over the fried chicken because it will taste better; that sitting on the couch won't feel as good as taking a walk. It can happen. Millions of people have done it. It's not magic. It's not that they are stronger than you, it's that they believed in themselves and wanted it more – maybe not totally, but just enough to get started. Once you get started, you'll realize you like the changes and just keep going.

When you see a runner on the road do you think, "I could never do that?" Without even knowing the person, we assume they are different. You need to get out of that mindset in order to be successful. The person you are judging may have had a more pathetic lifestyle and felt the same hopeless way as you at one time. So don't assume they are somehow different from you and then use it as an excuse for not pursuing your goals.

And if the runner passes you on a hill while you are struggling just to walk it, don't get discouraged. As I said before, the runner may have been like you at one time. No one is judging or comparing you. Most likely the runner is happy to see you doing the best you can.

I have a shameful memory that comes to mind when I take a jog. When I was about 19, an overweight party girl, I can remember throwing an empty beer can towards a runner along the road. This was not a typical reaction for me. I was not a mean person. So why did I act so horribly? What was going on inside of me? Was I taking my self-loathing behaviors out on someone else? Was I jealous because I thought I could never be that kind of person?

You need to believe that you can lose weight. But more importantly, you need to want to become a person that prefers to live differently than the way you do now. Stop thinking that changing the way you live is not normal for you or is impossible. You can change the way you behave and you will like it. You can do it and it's not a burden. Think about it. Have you ever heard anyone who has changed to a healthier lifestyle say his or her life was better before? We may believe it's because they lost weight but the weight loss is more the effect of the change, not the reason. Start visualizing that you can be a *better* you.

Change What You Want to Achieve

Don't start the journey with the primary (or only) goal of losing weight. Your goal is to feel better and live better. Nearly all people who lose weight permanently do so because they have changed the way they live their life.

When you focus only on your weight, you will always struggle because your lifestyle habits are what caused you to gain weight in the first place. Lifestyle change is the only way to "cure" your problem.

Redefine Your Life

If you make a decision to change and you want to change, you then need to create an environment for change. If your lifestyle does not invite healthy behaviors, then it's going to be difficult to change your behaviors. A lifestyle change involves much more than eating right and getting regular exercise. For lifetime results, you need to change how you live. Think about what aspects of your environment invite negative behaviors and then make changes in those areas to create a more positive environment. By positively changing your environment, you will set the stage for succeeding in the physical aspects of change (i.e., eating right and getting regular exercise).

Change Your Daily Routine

Change your style. Do things differently. Discover ways to make your life more interesting, more active, more exciting. Work towards a more active lifestyle. Create an environment for yourself that invites activity and healthy eating. Surround yourself with people who already are living or want to live a healthier lifestyle.

Make change a family thing. Convince your spouse to change with you. Start cooking together, take walks together, turn off the TV and go to bed earlier. Together.

Change the eating patterns of the entire family. I never understood women who go on diet programs like Jenny Craig. Mom gets to eat a pre-packaged dinner even though she just cooked dinner for the family. How successful (and resentful) is Mom going to be if she has to eat differently than the rest of the family?

If you don't own a pair of good sneakers, shame on you. If you never go out without your hair fixed and full make-up, chances are you would turn down an opportunity to get a little exercise because it would ruin your "look."

On some mornings, I don't shower until I exercise. Then I can't use "but I just took a shower" as an excuse for not doing it. When I do errands in my running shoes rather than heeled shoes, I find myself jogging from the parking lot into the store or just walking a little faster. The little extra movement you do throughout the day will burn more calories and the great feeling may stimulate you to do even more. The less you do, the less you want to do. The more you move, the more you want to move.

Find diversions to avoid unwise bad habits. Pay attention to your weak moments with food. Find the pattern and then find a diversion. In better weather, I go outside after dinner. Usually I end up talking to a neighbor and by the time I get in, it's almost time to get ready for bed. I completely missed the dreaded "dessert hour" when I'm most likely to give in to temptation. I have more energy than if I sat on the couch watching a *Seinfeld* rerun on TV. And more energy means less temptation.

Discover a New Passion

Find a passion other than food. My sister and I hypothesized that there is something in high mental energy that burns calories. We both find it easier to maintain our weight when we have a passion for something. I used to think a passion somehow speeds up metabolism. In reality I suppose the reason is that food takes second place to the stimulus. We actually have something more interesting to think about than food. It seems every time I made a significant change in my life – a new job, an escape from a bad relationship, a time-consuming project, etc. – I was able to lose weight without even trying.

If you are in a rut, find a new passion. Your choices are endless. Take flying lessons. Learn redecorating. Try scuba diving. Start a new job, even your own business. What have you always wanted to do, but never motivated yourself to do it?

Even if a new passion doesn't make you lose weight, you'll be having more fun so what do you have to lose?

Change Your Attitude Towards Food

Don't fight the desire for food. Don't feel guilty eating food. And whatever you do, don't avoid food in public and then have a secret affair with food when alone. It's okay to love food.

But, while we all love food, we must recognize its purpose. Its basic function is fuel for the body. Give your body a lot of crap and it runs like crap. Enjoy food, but remember its purpose and learn to enjoy giving your body food that is going to make it run well. If your body is running well, you will feel better.

Change What You Value as Being Good to Yourself

If you are overweight, being good to yourself may mean having potato skins and a bean and cheese burrito. But, think about it. If you do that often, how good is it, *really*? Do you feel more valuable by stuffing yourself and clogging your arteries? Do you feel good afterward? Think about changing what it means to be good to yourself. More importantly, allow yourself to deserve it.

Don't Be Selfless

Not being selfless doesn't mean you are selfish. Not being selfless allows you to care about yourself – to have some concern about your welfare. For many women, their needs fall behind everyone else's. We feel guilty taking time for ourselves.

You need personal time. When you don't get it you start to feel resentful, maybe even depressed. You will be a better mother, spouse, employee, significant other, whatever, if you take a little time for yourself.

Many of us use our selflessness as an excuse for not living a healthier lifestyle. We conclude we don't have time or someone or something else needs us more. We're not making an excuse for not exercising, it's just that many times we *allow* everything else to get in the way. Make time. You need it. You deserve it.

Think of a Positive Future

Many people start aging and sort of go into a coma. They do, but they don't dream. I don't mean dreaming as in winning a lottery ticket. I mean working towards a positive future.

For many, as we get older we dream through our children. We do for our children but not for ourselves. We are no longer a priority. Sometimes we feel the better part of our life is over. We lose our dreams and ourselves. We also lose connection with our bodies and minds. A great motivator for me to stay fit is to dream of the time when the kids are on their own and my husband and I can spend more time together: dreaming of playing golf and traveling. If I don't take care of myself now, I'll be too busy nursing my ailments to enjoy one of the best parts of my life!

Find Your Trigger

Remember the Subway restaurant commercial where the guy claimed he lost a lot of weight by eating Subway low-fat subs?

That's not why he lost all the weight, but it was a trigger for him. He found that eating a low-fat Subway sandwich instead of a Big Mac wasn't all that hard. Once he was successful at that change he was motivated to try other ways to positively change his life.

He was stimulated by his small success and it helped him recognize he could change and maybe change wasn't a bad thing. He lost a few pounds, felt better and it gave him the desire to do more.

Try to find your trigger. Find a new passion; experiment with different – healthier – foods; take time for yourself; rekindle a dream. Most success stories started with a spark that grew into a flame. If you discover the spark, don't blow it out, feed it.

Be Prepared for Setbacks

Even if you want to change and convince yourself you can change, be prepared for setbacks. When you feel you are ready for change, don't expect to always follow through with the change. Often we fail at changing our lifestyle because we confuse setbacks with failure. If you accept a setback as just a blip in the process, you won't give up and change back to your old way of thinking.

Most people who are successful at losing weight fail in the process. Recognizing that you don't have to be perfect to succeed will keep you on track. In fact, you can have daily setbacks and still succeed. The goal is to stay focused on the overall success. Accept setbacks as a part of the change process.

Even though I am liberated from my food and weight issues, I rarely meet my lofty expectations. I start every morning with the best intentions, but a day doesn't go by where I don't slip. Maybe I ate an extra handful of peanuts, or dipped into the ice cream a few times too many. But overall, I did all right. I had a big salad with grilled chicken for dinner, I resisted the cookies I nearly ate 20 minutes before dinner and I took a walk with my neighbor. No, I wasn't perfect, but I was a lot better than I used to be.

Then there are days I might have major setbacks. I can remember a bad PMS episode when I ate a large "boardwalk size" fries for dinner and then made a chocolate cake. I was in a feeding frenzy. I was a pig and I loved every minute of it – until it was over. Then I felt lousy. I had indigestion and my PMS symptoms were only worse.

The next morning I woke up and still felt terrible. I didn't feel terrible because I failed, I felt terrible because *I felt terrible!*

I didn't beat myself up out of guilt and failure, but I ate fewer calories and made healthy choices that day because I just wanted to feel better. If you focus on your temporary lapse as a failure you will likely return to your old way of thinking. "I can do it" turns into "I can't do it" and you give up.

I'm not perfect and I never expect to be. I think a binge is good for me every once in a while. It reminds me of what I'm not missing. Since I have taken the focus off of losing weight and consider how I feel, my binging is less frequent and less destructive. At least now I accept my weakness and I'm confident that one night of being out of control does not mean I am a bad, fat, weak person. It doesn't mean I have failed. There is a difference between failing and quitting. You can fail and still succeed, but if you quit, you've given up.

Are You Now Ready for Change?

Are you mentally ready to go on? Do you have a better understanding of your negative and destructive thinking and are you ready to take action?

- Have you made the decision to change?
- Are you convinced you can change?
- Are you realistic about your expectations?
- Are you ready to start living a healthy lifestyle?

If you can't positively answer these questions, don't bother going any further. Keep evaluating yourself. Keep working on changing your answer. Don't set yourself up for another failure by implementing the change process without the desire to change and the belief you can change.

If you are ready, it's time to get to the actual doing. It's time to learn how to eat by listening to your body's signals instead of your mind. And then it's time to discover The NEW You!

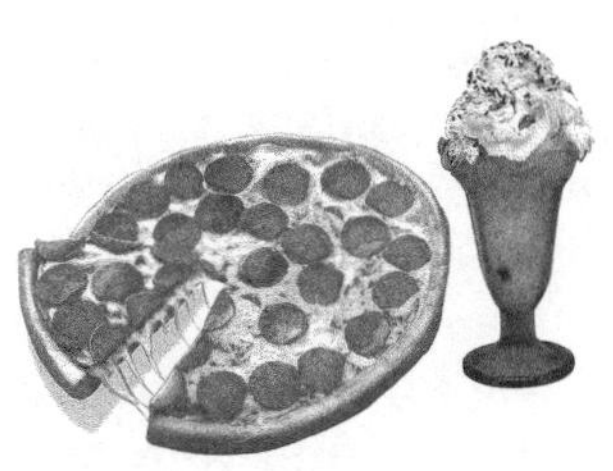

PART II
A New Way of Listening

Do you feel like you can't trust yourself with food? Do you feel confused by what to eat and how much to eat? Do you ever feel good after you splurge on a dessert? Do you avoid foods you crave because you think it's wrong to eat them? Do you ever stop to consider if you really even enjoy what you are eating? When was the last time you ate something without feeling guilty afterwards?

These feelings are caused by mental sabotage. The problem has gotten worse with today's obsession with food and dieting. We've been bombarded with so much information telling us what we can eat or shouldn't eat that we've stopped paying attention to what we really want or need. We question whether we're eating too much but ignore our bodies' signals that tell us we're full. We're told what foods we can have so we've stopped asking ourselves what we really want. And if we *do* ask, we conclude we can't have it anyway because we're not allowed to have it!

The struggle between the mind and body is powerful and our minds tend to win. Overeating, eating foods you really don't want and emotional eating are all calories consumed that your body really doesn't want or need, but your mind takes control and the result causes you to gain weight. It's not necessarily what you eat, but how much of it you eat. If you are ignoring what your body needs to be content, you will be discontented. In other words, eating wrong is when you are eating what your body doesn't really want.

Not listening is a big problem and contributes to food obsession. It causes us to eat what we don't want and eat more than we need. It contributes to bad habits. If you can learn to listen to your body and control bad habits that occur as a result of not listening, you will find maintaining or even losing weight effortless.

Unfortunately, listening to your body can be difficult, especially if you've been ignoring it for a long time. A New Way Of Listening will help you learn how to listen to your body's signals again.

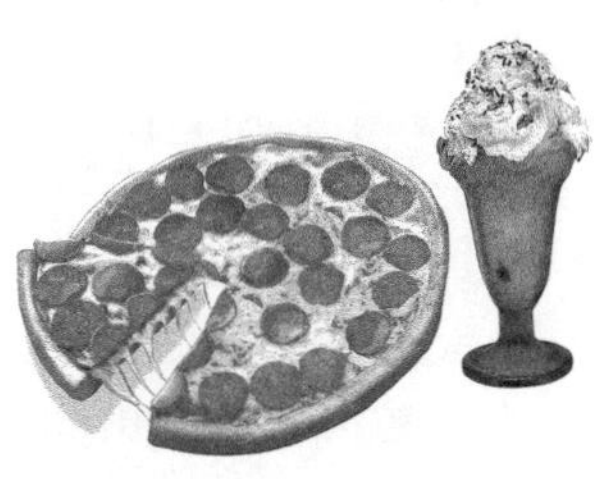

Chapter 12

STEP 5
Listen to Your Body, Not Your Mind

Have you ever chosen a garden salad at a restaurant but really wanted a sandwich? On the other hand, have you ever ordered the "colossal burger" when you really wanted a grilled chicken breast? When you decide to take an extra helping, do you make your decision based on the possible result on the scale? Do you make food decisions based on what you *think* you are supposed to eat?

If you've answered yes to any of the above questions, then you have allowed your mind to make your food decisions. But you're listening to the wrong signal. It's your body that should decide your food choices but you don't trust it anymore.

Moderation and balance in our eating habits are the keys to discovering a life without weight issues. Your body will naturally produce healthy eating habits, but you have to learn how to trust and listen to your body again. To listen to your body, you need to learn how to:

- Understand why you don't listen
- Make better choices for your health, not your looks
- Eat only what you crave
- Recognize what your body wants

- Get your body to listen
- Recognize the subtle difference between listening to your mind versus your body
- Trust yourself with food

If you can understand the subtle, but major difference between body listening and mind listening, you will never have a weight problem again.

Why We Don't Listen

Barry Sears talks about being "in the zone." You can put yourself "in the zone" by giving your body what it wants. If you listen to your body's wants and not your mind, your body will ask you for all the foods that it needs to put you in the zone and keep you there. And sometimes, it may want ice cream.

Your body is what should determine your need for food – what kind of food and how much food. Our body tells our brain. Unfortunately, outside influences have sabotaged our ability to listen to our bodies' signals. In today's environment, those influences have taken over and most of us hardly ever listen to what our bodies want anymore.

Food Confusion

A child can have a toy for six months and never play with it. But as soon as his friend picks it up, the child suddenly wants it. Not only does he want it, he'll yell, cry and even hit his friend to get it back. As soon as he gets his toy back, the child plays with it for 2 minutes and then doesn't touch it again until someone else takes it from him.

Because society has labeled food into categories of healthy and unhealthy (and the labeling keeps getting more and more confusing, limited and stringent) we are placing foods in categories of "can have" and "can't have." Just like the child with the toy, when it comes to food, we don't care about the "can have," we just want the "can't have."

Our society exacerbates the problem. High-fat, high-sugar foods are considered "yummy," while healthy foods are boring. I find it annoying when I sometimes have to justify my healthy food choices with other people. If I hover over the veggie tray and say, "No thank you," to the puff pastry, I'll hear, "Oh, you're being good today!" Or "You must be on a diet!" Some people don't even consider that I *prefer* to eat the carrots and pass on the cheesy pastry.

When we tell ourselves we can't have certain foods, we think we are missing out on something. We want it more. And when we give in to our intense mental desire we feel like we've done something wrong. Then the food becomes taboo. We start to develop a negative relationship with food and our food obsession gets worse.

To overcome your mental attitude towards food, you need to stop categorizing food. All food should be treated equally. All food is allowed. If you don't think about whether or not you can have the food, you can make a food decision by listening to what your body is saying.

Listening to Others

The problem with following a diet is it tells you what to eat. The problem gets bigger when you try to follow a diet where you have to restrict a whole category of food. When you diet, you mentally eat. You completely lose touch with what foods your body wants. Even if you did listen, you couldn't follow your body's advice because it would be against the diet rules!

With each new set of rules, your mental reaction to food takes over and you become confused. You stop recognizing your physical food needs. If you are a compulsive dieter, your view of food gets distorted. You are most likely obsessed with foods you can't have. Meanwhile you are eating foods you don't even want! You torture yourself by restricting the foods you want and by the end of the day relieve your suffering by giving in to your cravings. Then you feel guilty and out of control.

You are better off listening to your body rather than following a diet – even if you have trouble listening at first. At least you will be eating what you want.

I don't mean to say you should eat cookies and candy rather than go on a diet, but I think when we try to modify our diets too much we stop naturally eating what we want and only react to what we can or shouldn't eat. Then we feel deprived and become obsessed.

Work on eating healthier, but try to include foods you really enjoy. Don't torture yourself; don't deprive yourself. And remember, there is no food that you "can't have."

I Chose to Ignore the Signals

A good example of when I used to ignore my body's needs (with my old behaviors) occurred at restaurants. Looking over the menu, some of the healthier entrées looked pretty good to me, but my eyes would steer back to the ribs and fried onion strings, the "baddest" entrée on the menu. It was calling me. I was on the edge, not knowing what to do. Should I have the chicken kabobs, the ribs, chicken kabobs . . . What?

A hovering waitperson only compounded my problems. "May I take your order?" she asks impatiently. I replied: "Chiiiccc . . . er make mine the rib platter please and add some potato skins!" In the end I would choose one of the most fattening options and then to make sure I had enough, I'd order more!

No sooner did the meal arrive than I would look at the plate and think, "My gosh, look at all this greasy food. I shouldn't do this!" I would relish the hot, crispy, onion strings, get my hands gooey with ribs and within 5 minutes of ravenous eating I would look at the remains and get sick. The crisp onion strings turned soggy; the coagulated fat on the ribs grossed me out. I felt fat and guilty at the choice I made.

In the end, I didn't think, "Gee, that was really good." I said to myself, "Why did I do that! I really wanted the chicken kabobs! And these potato skins, why the hell did I order those!" I'd go to bed with heartburn and a guilty conscience and I'd swear I'd never do it again.

My body didn't want the ribs and onion strings, but my mind took over and I followed. So did I learn anything? No. The next time I would do the same thing. I wasn't listening to what my body wanted. My mind was controlling my decision by some preconceived notion that only greasy, fattening foods tasted good; that somehow I was missing out on something if I didn't eat the greasy, fattening food.

So why do we feel that way? Why don't we choose the foods our bodies really want? Why do we believe we want the fattening, greasy food when, 10 minutes after we eat, our bodies start protesting! Why can't we learn from our mistakes? How many times do we have to feel like crap after we eat before we learn it's the crappy food?

I mean, think about it. Do healthier options really taste bad? Have you ever wished you had gotten the greasy platter after you've eaten the healthier option? Well, unless it was a poorly prepared or tasteless option, for most of us the answer is no.

Let's clarify that the "healthier" option I'm referring to doesn't mean low calorie. It doesn't mean you have to eat cottage cheese and peaches or a salad with low-calorie dressing. It simply means choosing foods that contain more nutrients, less fat, fewer calories or more protein than your current diet. And it means consuming them in moderation. Our body craves healthy foods but we keep ignoring these intense urgings.

Typically, if you eat few vegetables, lots of high-fat foods and mostly starchy carbohydrates, simply choosing better foods will make you feel better and help you eat fewer calories.

Now when I eat out, I frequently choose healthier foods because I prefer them. However, after a game of golf or working out in the yard all day, a cheeseburger and a double-dip homemade ice cream cone might taste really good. I may chow down a thousand calories but my stomach agrees with the choice. And my body agrees it needed all those calories. So I don't feel guilty afterward.

Make Better Choices for Health, Not Looks

Many of us decide that if we aren't willing to sacrifice ourselves to obtain the perfect body, we might as well give up and not do anything about it. We feel it's not worth being healthier if we can't look good. We feel cheated because we don't look like the lucky two percent of the population who have "perfect" genes so we just say screw it and stop caring.

We don't seem to care how eating poorly and gaining weight makes us feel terrible and eventually can kill us. I don't mean look terrible, I mean *feel* terrible: sluggish, tired, unhappy or even depressed. We don't consider what our bodies are feeling. We don't consider the negative impact bad health habits have on our lives. Our minds are in a state of hopelessness based on the mirror. I believe if every "body" was exactly the same no matter what we ate and all food contained the same amount of calories, we would naturally eat a well-balanced diet.

Your Focus Is Everything

Changing your mindset can change how you view food. When you're focused on weight gain or body image, giving into a decadent piece of cheesecake results in feelings of guilt and weakness. When you focus on how you feel, rather than the repercussions of the scale, you can make a choice based on your body's wants and needs. The result is satisfaction and enjoyment of food.

Let's face it, eating takes about 5 minutes, but the recriminating aftermath of eating what your body doesn't want or need can last for hours. During those hours, you might feel overly full, guilty, and yet, still craving something. What's worse is the negative feelings only escalate with each poor decision. Pretty soon you feel unable to control yourself and you spiral downward. You feel hopeless; you feel addicted.

By making choices based on your body's needs you can enjoy a splurge nearly every day as long as your body has been fed what it needs. If you have had a balance of foods over the course of the day, have not overeaten and have moved your body, a serving of your favorite dessert will not only taste good, but it will digest easily and you will enjoy it more. Your body doesn't respond negatively and you don't feel you have to serve penance afterward.

How Thin People Do It

When I discuss this book with people who don't have weight issues, they don't get it. "I eat whatever I want," they say, "I just watch what I eat." We interpret that to mean they eat what we eat or more and don't gain weight.

But most likely they don't eat as much as you. And if they do, they are still only eating as much as their body needs. They generally don't overeat. Think about it. *If you really stopped eating when you were full and you only ate what you really needed, would you have a weight problem?*

People without weight issues may have weak moments now and then, but generally they don't fear eating. They don't have an emotional struggle with food. The majority of them are active people who may have their nightly ice cream or piece of pie. Many aren't thin or aesthetically fit, but they are within a healthy range. They don't think, "Gee, I *should* eat this or I *have to* exercise." They are active. It might not be from 30 minutes on a treadmill, but maybe gardening, housecleaning, tennis, golf, playing ball in the street with the kids or just walking. People with healthy lifestyles naturally seem to enjoy activities requiring body movement. They aren't resistant to it.

People who unconsciously live a healthy lifestyle are not screwed up by body image. They are not obsessed with their bodies or the whole weight thing and so they aren't obsessed with food.

They don't consider any food forbidden but they typically eat a balanced diet. They eat what their body wants, they stop when it's full and when they're feeling a little stiff or sluggish, they go for a walk. Their bodies may not be perfectly proportioned, but they generally feel good about themselves.

And isn't that what matters? As I've said before, there will always be those who appear better looking than you. So for now, don't focus on how you look; pay more attention to how you feel. You can't compare yourself, your body image, with anyone else. You have a unique body.

Becoming One of "Those" People

All my life I thought I couldn't be a person without weight issues. I was different from them. Even when I lost weight, I thought I could never be released from my obsession. Ironically, the thinner I got, the more obsessed I became. Food always controlled me.

Discovering I had the ability to overcome my obsession – to be one of "those" people – was an incredible awakening for me. Listening to my body's wants instead of my mind; making choices based on how I feel, rather than the mirror, liberated me. Now food is my friend. I can enjoy eating without worrying.

If food becomes a reflection of your body, you aren't focusing on food's importance. Food is fuel for your body. Your body needs good fuel. Your body reacts negatively to too much food. You don't feel good if you eat too much, so don't eat any more than you need.

If you focus on your body's response to the food you are about to eat, you will likely find it easier to control your weight gaining habits. To do that, you have to push away all the feelings of sacrifice, hopelessness and unrealistic expectations, and think more about your health, your improved energy levels and your general well-being.

Eat Only What Your Body Craves

Virtually all foods are comprised of but three nutrients: protein, fat and carbohydrate. Your body needs all three components and it will crave them if it doesn't get them.

If you watch a young child (before his mind is corrupted by commercials and exposure to junk food), you will notice that as long as the child is not denied any food, the child will naturally have a fairly well-balanced diet. The day after Halloween or Easter, my kids want nothing but meat and vegetables for dinner. If we've had meat and vegetables for three days in a row, they want pizza.

For generations most people's diets were moderate. We didn't pay attention to how much fat or processed food we ate. We didn't have sugar addicts or carbohydrate addicts. Food was enjoyed, but our lives didn't revolve around it. People had breakfast, lunch, dinner and snack. Your mother made you eat your fruits and vegetables, but she'd have homemade cookies ready when you got home from school (but you were only allowed two so you wouldn't spoil your dinner!). Dinner didn't come from a drive-thru; it was more like pot roast, carrots and potatoes. We ate until we were full and if we started to feel our belt tightening, we'd forego that second helping or skip the pie for a week or two.

Diet books have gotten to the point where they have labeled just about every food as "bad" for you. With this kind of information being thrown at us, no wonder our minds aren't listening to what our bodies want. Everyone is telling us not to listen! We are told that our cravings are really just an addiction, a vitamin deficiency or a weakness. So we go on diets that eliminate certain foods and when we have a craving we drive ourselves nuts trying to do anything but eat what we want to eat. So we eat this and that and a little more of this and, if you are lucky you'll stop there. Instead of avoiding your craving, you end up eating stuff you don't even want.

How I Resolved My Craving Problem

When I tried to eliminate certain foods from my diet, I tried to give up my favorite treat, chocolate. There are times that I crave chocolate. Well, really I crave it almost every day. It seems after dinner I just have to have some in order to feel satisfied. So since I couldn't have, for example, M&M's (one of my favorites) I'd have alternatives: yogurt, cottage cheese, fruit, cereal, oatmeal, or fat-free ice cream. I'd try to fool myself into satisfying my craving. I didn't give in to the M&M's but I admit I was eating more calories trying to eat "around" my craving for M&M's.

Mentally saying "no" to your cravings only makes you want them more. I tried to avoid my chocolate cravings for years. Now, I just eat the M&M's.

I had to learn to control how many of them I ate. I had to resist sitting in front of the TV with the whole bag. After years of staying away from the M&M's or feeling weak or bad when I would give in to them, I found it was easier and more enjoyable to have the M&M's but control how many of them I ate.

This was difficult at first because I didn't trust myself. I thought I couldn't control the quantity. I thought I was an addict. It took practice, but it didn't take long for me to adjust and, while I still have the urge to methodically eat half the bag (once in a while I still do), I usually resist.

I plan my indulgence. First of all, I wait until I have time to enjoy my indulgence. I'll grab a cup of decaf and measure out a serving, and I savor every one. Sometimes I'll go back and get some more, but I'm always conscious of how much I eat even if I eat more than I should. I never throw handfuls in my mouth like most people do. I might eat about 350 calories of them on some nights, but that's at least what I was eating in cereal and other low-fat or fat-free foods. And when I've had my treat, I am satisfied.

Looking back, when I used to avoid chocolate I just couldn't stop eating. I'd pour a bowl of cereal, at least two servings, and when I was through, I'd pull out the fat-free or sugar-free ice cream and then eat more cereal out of the box. And when I was done, I was full but I still wasn't content. I really just wanted the M&M's and now that I eat them, even in smaller quantities, I'm satisfied. I enjoy what I am eating and usually I consume fewer overall calories.

Eating M&M's doesn't make us fat. Eating too many M&M's does. Eating too much of anything makes us fat. Be aware of how much you are eating, but if you crave chocolate, eat chocolate. Just don't eat too much of it. It's not easy to train yourself to stop overeating the foods we love, but the alternative – not eating them at all – is harder to do and less satisfying.

Think Before You Act

Try to go beyond what your mind is saying about the food you are about to eat. Pay more attention to how you feel. Listen to what your body is saying. Are you hungry? Are you full? Does what you are eating taste good? Is it what you wanted? Immediately, you may conclude that you are always hungry and you are never full and everything tastes good. I don't believe it. I believe that's what you think, but I don't believe that's how you really feel. If you can figure out the difference, you will never have a weight problem again.

How Can You Recognize What and How Much Your Body Wants?

If your mind has been taking over your food responsibility for a long time, it may be difficult to know what your body is telling you to eat.

Listen to yourself. If you really listen, you will hear a voice that says, "I've had enough." If you think things through you will know what the answer is to that second helping, handful, slice, piece, whatever it is. Instead of thinking, "I'm not full enough," tell yourself, "I don't want to get up from the table with regrets. I want to enjoy what I've eaten." Sure, once in a while you might overindulge, but the frequency and the amount needs to be in control.

It's okay to eat pizza, chocolate, anything you crave, just don't eat so much of it and eat it as part of a healthy diet. In other words, most of the time you should be eating good stuff like vegetables, lean protein, fibrous foods, calcium rich foods, etc. But, it's okay to treat yourself, even on a daily basis, to some fun foods. You just need to learn to stay in control. Once you get some control of your food intake, your "bad" won't be as "bad" as it used to be, yet, the mental experience will be the same.

I believe that without distorted mental thinking, our bodies would naturally send us signals about what to eat, when to eat and how much to eat. But we can't just turn off those thoughts and steer ourselves toward more enlightened, more responsive thinking.

STEP 5: Listen to Your Body, Not Your Mind

Here are some ways to help you listen:

Don't Eat What You Don't Want

How much food do you put in your mouth every day that you don't even want? If you get a lot of your calories cleaning off your kid's plate or choosing inferior tasting foods to save a calorie, you need to refocus on what food means to you. Would you rather eat the last few spoonfuls of your kid's cold macaroni and cheese or save the calories for something you really want? Would you rather end up eating three servings of fat-free ice cream after a weak moment while on a deprivation diet or anticipate having a homemade brownie after a good long walk?

When we try to avoid foods we desire, we can sometimes give in to foods we don't want and then still feel deprived because we didn't get the food we really wanted! We end up eating the same amount of calories or more only we spend them on less appetizing or desirable foods and we still feel guilty eating them! The problem with many diets is they tell you what to eat, some of which your body may not want at the time.

Put Taste in Perspective

Some may say, I do listen, but the food tastes too good to stop! That's what you may think, but if you don't put arbitrary limits on the kind of foods you can eat, you can experience any taste you want. Our minds, not our tongues, control much of the desire for certain foods and the taste of those foods. If you allow your body to control what you desire to eat, you will find that if it doesn't want candy, it doesn't want candy no matter how good you *think* it tastes!

Visual Control

Sometimes we give in to visual desire. For example, a "beautiful" dessert or an elaborate fried appetizer can be very enticing, but sometimes the taste can be disappointing compared to the visual. And we eat it anyway. The next time you give in to a yummy "looking" cake, think about how it tastes. Maybe it doesn't taste as good as you thought it would. The reality might be that the cake is dry and the icing tastes like sweetened plastic. Pay attention to how food *really* tastes.

Use Your Sense of Taste to Determine What You Really Crave

Do you want something sweet, salty or crunchy? Are you just eating whatever is convenient and not what you really want? I have found myself eating 300 calories of crackers when I'm not even hungry and still have a taste for something only to find out I really wanted a crunchy apple. I love a good apple, but I still always seek out the crackers or other less nutritious, higher calorie alternatives unless I take a minute to think about what I really want; what would satisfy me.

Try the Healthier Alternative First

If you are in doubt about what it is you really want, try the healthier alternative first. Don't forbid yourself from having the food you crave, but make sure you know what you are craving before you eat it. Is it a mental craving or a physical craving? It's easier to turn off healthy cravings than unhealthy ones so more than likely you don't know because you are mentally resisting the healthier option. I can't tell you how many times I've opened the refrigerator thinking, "I want something, what is it?" I immediately think I want cookies or crackers or chips but I know now that if I have to think about it, that's probably not it. Nothing else in the refrigerator excites me. I decide to pick at some leftover cantaloupe, and, to my surprise, it tastes so good! I realized it was fruit I was craving. But I was resisting the fruit because of my old thinking that fruit is boring.

How to Get Yourself to Listen to Your Body

So how do you start knowing what your body wants? You won't know what your body wants until you shoo away all the mental reasons for your food choices. It worked for me. Once I stopped thinking so much, I was able to listen.

I took my mind out of the equation. I stopped obsessing about what I ate. I started to eat whole fat ice cream and pizza with real cheese again. I stopped trying to frantically work off excess calories I might have eaten that day by running endlessly on a treadmill. After so many years, it was hard to do. I didn't believe I could trust my body to tell me what and how much to eat. I still believed I was incapable of control and I was a bit frightened at the outcome. I was afraid of turning into an overweight couch potato again.

To my surprise, it never happened. I also found exercise to be easier and more fun. Today I exercise not because I'm trying to burn off extra calories, but because I feel better afterward, especially if I have overeaten.

I allow myself to eat all the "bad" foods. Although generally, I prefer eating vegetables, lean meats and whole grain breads because they taste better! If I have a healthy dinner and a good dose of exercise for the day, I eat ice cream. And I'm not talking a half-cup of ice cream; I'm talking more like one or even two cups if I had physically worked hard that day. On a Friday night, I'll have pizza, if I want it. But, it usually only tastes good if I have eaten healthy the rest of the week. The freedom from guilt makes it taste all the better.

The Subtle But Major Difference

How we think about the food we eat is critical, yet the difference is subtle. If you change your attitude about food, you can allow your body to respond and hear the signals. Like changing "I have to" to "I want to," changing how we feel about the food itself is critical. It's hard to explain, so let me give you an example of my changed reaction to food.

Changed View Equals Success

When I restricted certain foods from my diet, I was never satisfied. I was always searching for something to appease my craving. I'd eat everything except what I truly wanted. The result was that I'd either eat too many calories in foods I really didn't want or I'd break down and eat everything. The result was overeating, dissatisfaction and guilt. I became even more obsessed with food, especially the foods I couldn't have.

Once I got rid of the obsession and changed how I felt about food, my whole approach to eating changed from deprivation and sacrifice to enjoyment.

Before

I remember one time I was at a party and there were lots of great desserts (always my favorite). I avoided them all evening. I would walk by and say to myself, "No, you can't have that." As the night went on, the goodies on the table became more and more vivid. I would avoid walking by them, but then I'd find myself purposely standing right above them. I would think about them when I was in the next room. One dessert, in particular, was dense whipped cream strawberry shortcake that looked so beautiful. I could smell a hint of the fresh strawberries as I passed by.

As the evening went on, I ate a lot of other things as a diversion until I was quite full. Then I finally snuck a small cookie or two, justifying it by saying, "It's only a little thing. I'll work it off tomorrow." As long as I avoided the cake, I would be okay.

When the end of the evening approached, a few of us girls remained in the kitchen right in front of the table of desserts. We were talking and I was weakening until I couldn't stand it anymore. I finally looked over and said, "If I don't have a piece of that cake, I'm going to kill myself!"

They all laughed and said, "Go ahead, like you really have to worry about your weight." Well, that's all I needed to hear. I broke down and took a small piece. Four bites, it was gone. The desire for the second piece was even greater than the first. I took a second, larger piece. I ate that. The urge didn't stop. I started eating the brownies, the little pecan pastries (I don't even like them that much) and halfway through the frenzy the guilt set in but not for long. The old standby, "What the hell, you already blew it," applied so I ate and ate until I couldn't take another bite. To top it off, I ended up taking some of the shortcake home so I could continue my torture the next day.

After

When I trained myself to listen to my body, my whole outlook on food changed. It wasn't a major effort; I just changed my view of food. Instead of food being "good" or "bad"; "I can have", "I can't have"; deprivation or guilt, my obsession with food has gone away. All food is treated equally. Nothing is taboo. I can have any food I want, but I choose my food wisely. If I listen to what my body wants I can enjoy the food I choose. No guilt, no ravenous eating binges and, most importantly, no regrets.

Let me give you the same example of the party, giving my new way of dealing with food.

Let's say I'm at the party and the same desserts are there. I walk by them and say, "Wow, I've got to try some of those desserts, especially that cake!" I don't mind not eating them until later because I am enjoying hors d'oeuvres and wine. During the party, I walk by the desserts and they aren't calling me, they aren't dancing in front of my eyes, they are just there. While I'm eating hors d'oeuvres, I eat a little less because I know I'm going to have dessert and I want to enjoy it so I don't want to be too full. Then, when I'm ready, I get a cup of decaf, look everything over and take the dessert that is my favorite or I'm most in the mood for, regardless of the calories. I take a plate, sit down, and enjoy it. Sure, I still get the urge to eat more but as long as I stop and consider how I'll feel afterwards, I only need a little willpower to say, "Enough!" I usually find that once I've had what I really wanted, I'm usually too full to eat anymore. I don't feel deprived and I don't feel guilty.

Comparing the Subtle Differences

So what was the difference?

- First of all, instead of thinking, "I can't have that," I said, "I'm going to have that!" The decision was made. Therefore, waiting for it was easy. I didn't give the food a chance to taunt me all night.
- Then, instead of eating a lot throughout the night, I ate a little less knowing I was going to eat the dessert and I didn't want other, less important foods to spoil the fun.
- I listened to my body's signals to tell me what and when to eat instead of what I was supposed to eat or what I shouldn't eat.
- Because I wasn't caught up in an obsessive frenzy, I ate only the dessert I truly wanted and stopped before I got overly full. (I realize now that it spoils the pleasure).
- I ate exactly what I wanted instead of eating "around my craving."

Learning to Trust Yourself with Food

Probably the hardest part of implementing your "listening" skills is the fear of not being able to control yourself with food. How could it be that easy? I didn't believe it either, until I tried it.

For 30 years I was obsessed with food, dieting and the scale. After I threw in the towel, I discovered my problem wasn't a physical weakness for food, but a mental food obsession caused by my fear of food and lack of faith in myself. Once I stopped dieting and obsessing, controlling my food intake and my weight became easy. For the past few years I have given in to my nightly chocolate splurge and enjoyed pizza night without regrets, and I have never felt better about myself. I started to trust myself with food and accepted my imperfect body. I was liberated and it closed a long and arduous chapter in my life.

An article in the *Ladies' Home Journal* (July 2001) mirrors my success and conclusion of the benefits of *not* dieting and allowing all foods back into your life. The article concerned a study that followed three chronic dieting women. They were asked to eat everything they wanted for a month. The result? Not only did they not gain weight, they also changed their attitudes about food. The article pointed out:

> *"Most women in this country, no matter what their weight, live in a perpetual purgatory of diet vigilance. We count every calorie, pass up enticing treats and deprive ourselves of entire segments of the food pyramid. But what would happen if we stopped denying ourselves? Would we really feed on nothing but pizza and candy bars (ironic comparison, isn't it)?*

Interviews of the three women gave incredibly similar experiences. Let me quote a few paragraphs from one woman's diary:

> Week 4: *I've been more motivated to exercise and eat right just to feel better. I've been really wanting to eat fruit, again; not to lose weight, but because my body desires it.*
>
> Results: *I lost one pound! This experiment has shown me that denying myself certain foods was only making me binge. Now I plan to stick with healthy foods that I really enjoy. I think I'll be a much more sensible eater, but I'll still eat my chocolate!*

Success Is as Easy As . . .

Listening to your body is not easy at first, but it's a lot easier than dieting. Just remember what I told you:

- Don't give up any food you enjoy
- Eat only what you want
- Think about what you want and choose your food wisely
- Think about how you'll feel if you eat more
- Eat slowly. Acknowledge and enjoy the food you eat

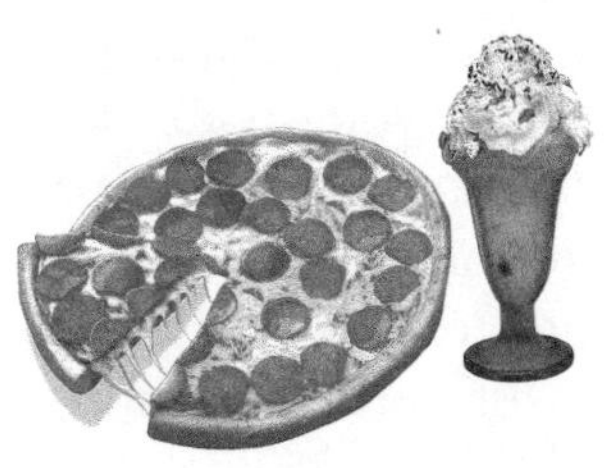

Chapter 13

STEP 6
How to Control Your Bad Habits

Bad habits are another reason we don't listen to our bodies and a big reason we have weight problems. Bad habits cause us to eat too much. Bad habits have more to do with how we eat our food rather than what we eat. If you can identify and control bad habits, you will eat less. It's a conscious awareness of what you are doing and taking simple steps to change. In order to do this, you have to identify your bad habits and then move towards overcoming them – or at least controlling them.

In the process of resolving my eating problems, I found I had bad habits and discovered methods to control them. You can discover and learn to control your own.

Eating Too Fast

Eating too fast causes overeating. Many times we overeat because the enjoyment of eating the food is over too fast and we want more because we aren't mentally satisfied.

Eating slower can reduce your caloric intake without effort because you experience the same taste pleasure with less consumption. Also by eating slower, your body has time to acknowledge it's full and you will reach the same satisfaction level with less food.

Here's an experiment. When you are eating, pay attention to *how* you are eating. When you swallow, is there so much food going down that it feels lumpy in your throat? Is the next forkful in your mouth ready to follow? At the same time, are you ready to shovel in still another forkful?

Now, try eating slower. How do you do that? Put less food on your fork or spoon. Chew your food more so that when you swallow, it feels more comfortable. Then, take another bite *after you swallow*. Make the process two steps, not three. One forkful is digested before the next forkful comes in. If you are eating with someone, stop the process while talking and **don't talk with your mouth full!** You'd think I wouldn't have to say this, but I observe a lot of people doing it and it's really quite disgusting!

Eating slower takes practice. If you find yourself "woofing" down food, stop yourself. Slow down. Enjoy it! If you keep reminding yourself to slow down, eventually you will naturally start eating slower and you will enjoy food more. It really works!

Overeating

There are times when I am out to dinner, at Grandma's or at a party with great food and I overeat. I don't feel good afterward, but I made a decision to overeat because the food and environment was a special occasion. While food should be enjoyed, every meal should not be a special occasion to overeat. I like to compare it to drinking at a party. A lot of us get tipsy or overindulge in alcohol at a party. You pay the price the next day and tell yourself you'll never do it again. And for a while, most of us won't, but eventually we slip and do it again. However, if the alcohol overindulgence becomes chronic and consumption increases in amount and frequency, it becomes "a problem."

The overeating I am referring to is when we chronically overeat. Most of my life I was a chronic overeater. We aren't satisfied until we are so full we are uncomfortable. It's the justification that our eating switch doesn't seem to turn off. But our switch does turn off, we just don't listen to it. I am not cured of my bad eating habits, but I have learned to control them. Here are a few control methods that work for me. Maybe they can help control your bad habits.

STEP 6: How to Control Your Bad Habits

Decide Who's In Charge

Before you go for the extra helping, ask yourself what is making you want more. Think about whether your mind is at work or your body. If your body doesn't answer, think about how you'll feel afterward if you keep eating. Will you be sluggish? Will you be uncomfortable and suffer from indigestion? Will you mentally beat yourself up? Take a second to ask yourself, "Do I even want this?"

Stop Eating for a Second

If you're at the stage where your body should be saying, "I'm full," but you're still shoveling in food, stop eating and look at your plate just for a few seconds. Stare at it. If you look at it closely enough and if you've really had enough, you might find that it really isn't very appealing (remember the ribs and onion strings?). Now, if you aren't satisfied yet, that shouldn't happen. But if you are full and are just eating because . . . stop and think about what you are doing.

My husband and I were having dinner together. I made a spicy Italian dish and we were enjoying a glass of wine and conversation while lingering over our meal. My husband got up from the table and took a second helping. I followed him and took another helping myself. As I sat down and ate a few bites, I looked down and stared at the food and thought, "I don't want this." I jokingly referred to this book and said, "My body doesn't want this. My mind just thinks it does." My husband, who's tired of me being on my soapbox, quipped back in his deadpan voice, "I know, that's why I have to eat it real fast so my body doesn't get a chance to object until I'm already done." He's sooooo funny!

Eat What's On Your Plate First

Overeating can occur when we don't acknowledge the food that is on our plate. While we're eating what's on our plate, we are anticipating what we are going to eat next. I was guilty of this behavior. I discovered the problem when I took the time to stop and think about how I was eating. I recognized that I was rushing to finish my plate. I didn't have to go anywhere. I had time to enjoy my meal. So why was I doing it? I concluded I wanted to finish what I had so I could have some more!

The next time you are gobbling up dinner, ask yourself why you are in a hurry to eat more calories than you need.

Walk Away for a Minute

I spend a lot of my time writing and I'm alone all day. As a mental break I love to watch *All My Children* with my lunch (laugh if you want but I'm comfortable with it). I know I'm breaking my own eating rules, but I never said I was perfect. I'll fix myself something and, practicing what I preach, I try to pay attention and enjoy my food but with one eye on the TV. When I'm done (especially if the show isn't over) I want more. I admit to myself I'm not hungry, but I want to eat more. Instead of saying, "No you can't" I give myself an option. I'm going to turn off TV and go fold the laundry, or make a phone call or something else. After, if I still want "whatever" I can have it. Most of the time it works and I can go for three hours without even thinking about food again.

It Tastes Too Good to Stop!

Another big excuse for overeating is because the food tastes too good to stop. But does it really? I mean if you eat it slowly and savor the sights, smells and tastes of your food, isn't that enough enjoyment? If you are giving your body the food it really wants and you can enjoy eating all foods, the taste issue will be placed in a reasonable perspective. If it tastes so good, then why are we in such a hurry to eat it?

Don't Eat on the Cheap

Cheap food is usually fat laden and abundant. Instead of once a week dinner visits at a low-priced restaurant with mediocre high-calorie foods, save your money for better food at a more upscale restaurant. Upscale restaurant food is generally healthier and tastes much better. You "experience" food rather than just eat it.

Keep Food Less Accessible

When eating informally, don't put the food on the table. Have the family fix a plate and bring it to the table. It takes more effort and thought to get up from the table and get a second helping. Also, when it's right there, we tend to pick at it. I used to only put a basket of bread on the table until I realized, while second helpings were reduced, everyone was eating more bread! Now, the only thing I keep on the table with casual dinners is a big bowl of salad.

If you have any food open on the counter (cookie jars, cakes, pies, etc.) you are at risk of noshing on it. Put it away. "Out of sight, out of mind."

Minimize Reading, TV or "Hot Issue" Conversation While Eating

Get into the habit of shutting off the TV at dinnertime. At least take your nose out of the newspaper for a moment and pay attention to the fact that *you are* eating. You may find that by paying attention to your meals, you enjoy them more and consume less. Dinner is a good time for family conversation but if you are arguing or nagging or venting about your bad day at work, no one is paying attention to the bounty that they should be thankful for. Meals should be enjoyed and acknowledged.

Emotional Eating

I don't consider emotional eating a habit. It's a psychological issue. Emotional eating was discussed in Step 1: Valuing Ourselves Through Food. However, the response to your emotions can become a habit.

I mentioned earlier emotional eating is a trancelike experience. The next time you emotionally eat, try to come out of your eating trance long enough to recognize your actual eating behavior. While you may still emotionally eat you might be able to minimize gluttonous eating.

Fighting Back

Most of us are guilty of emotional eating from time to time. I am. I have reduced the frequency by valuing myself but, on occasion, it still happens. I *allow* it to happen. But I minimize the damage by recognizing what I am doing.

For example, I'm suffering from PMS symptoms and have the urge to wallow in my emotions. By allowing myself to emotionally eat, I don't deny my actions. Instead I have a constructive binge. I acknowledge that I have the ice cream container and a spoon in hand. As I dig in, ready to wallow in self-pity, I analyze my actions. I try to figure out the reason I am doing it. Usually, I am overreacting to little things that somehow seem overwhelming at the time. Most of the time I feel pretty good about myself, so I accept that my feelings are only temporary. Once I gain perspective, I view the ice cream differently. I come out of the trance, put the ice cream back and walk away without regrets – even if I did just eat 400 calories. At least I didn't eat 1,000!

By allowing, analyzing and redirecting your actions, you become your own therapist. You are the best one to figure out why you are eating.

To minimize the damage of the eating you do, look at the binge food. Be creative with it. See if you can do something besides eat it. I've discovered the emotional action is sometimes more important than the actual eating. Getting back to the ice cream, while my head is in the container, I try to play with the food to minimize eating it. I stir it, poke at it, or make designs with it. Even if I have to throw the ice cream away because I have turned it into mush, at least I didn't throw it in my stomach. We are taught not to waste food, but if eating it results in weight gain, the food is better off in the trash.

Mindless Eating

Many of us eat without even thinking. We aren't hungry; we aren't craving something – we just eat. I can go all day completely content with moderate eating and looking forward to a nice dinner. But when my husband walks through the door, he sets off my eating alarm.

He's hungry. And while telling me about his day he starts snacking. First he opens the peanuts; then he gets out the cheese and crackers. And when he starts, I start. I start grabbing a few peanuts, a few crackers and before you know it I've eaten about 300 calories of stuff.

In the old days, I would have been upset because I had to make up those "bad" 300 calories and would have to force myself to eat less for the rest of the day fearing I might gain a pound. Nowadays, when I am guilty of this, I'm still mad at myself for mindlessly eating, for a different reason. I wasn't going to be very hungry for dinner. Remember when your mother used to say you're going to spoil your appetite? I do. If I waste my calories (my physical desire for food) on junk, I'll lose the enjoyment of the dinner I'm so looking forward to.

How do you control mindless eating? Here are some things I try to do with some success.

STEP 6: How to Control Your Bad Habits

Pay Attention to Why and When You Are Eating

You should be hungry for breakfast, lunch and dinner, and a light snack in between is okay (if you are hungry). But if you are grabbing a cookie or a handful of chips several times a day you need to stop and ask yourself why you are doing it and if you are enjoying it. If you question everything you are about to put in your mouth, you will eat less.

Stop Eating

Once you've decided that your body doesn't really need anything, let alone a cookie, just stop! Don't laugh! I know you're thinking, "What, are you crazy? If I could stop, I would!" Well, you can. But it has to be a conscious decision. There are times when I will open the drawer, take out a cookie, have a bite and then throw it away because I took a moment to say, "Why am I eating this?"

Expect that you aren't always going to be successful. But see if you can at least stop yourself a few times a day, a week, and keep trying. Once I became conscious of what I was doing, I stopped.

Control the Damage

I think most of us mindlessly eat from time to time. You just feel like munching even though you aren't hungry. If you feel compelled to do this, try to stick with less damaging foods.

The desire for the process of eating is different than craving a certain food. If you just want to do the action, try alternatives that won't bust your waistline. Light popcorn or stick pretzels with mustard, for example. Your munching goes a lot further.

Getting back to my before dinner actions with my husband, a great way to minimize the damage is to add a bag of precut carrots to the snack assortment. If I can alternate some carrots with the crackers, I've controlled the damage.

This works well at parties as well. I try to hang around the veggie tray and sample only one or two high-fat hors d'oeuvres instead of six.

Stay Out of the Kitchen

The more you are around food, the harder it is to resist. This is hard for me because I work at home. I have clear vision of my kitchen from where I write. Nowadays, the kitchen is Grand Central Station for family and friends. Our kitchen is large, inviting and directly connected to the family room. The temptation is always there because the food is always there.

Because I can't stay out of the kitchen, I have trained myself with some success to mentally disassociate food and kitchen. As I said before, food is all around us, now more than ever. We can't make it go away, so we have to find ways to live with it. It's working most of the time (as long as I keep the goodies off the counter) and I take a moment to decide if I really do want something to eat.

Go to Bed Earlier

The family often goes upstairs around nine o'clock. We may not go to bed, but we settle in. My husband and I find that we are most vulnerable to eating at night – even when we aren't hungry. Once you're in the bedroom, it's a lot easier to stay away from food (and maybe you'll find something else to crave in the bedroom rather than the kitchen!).

Besides, many of us are not getting enough sleep. Do you get eight hours a night? You should but it's hard when life is so hectic. Adequate sleep will help you stay in control of food. When you are tired, you are more vulnerable to overeating and picking. Your willpower diminishes because you are too tired to fight your temptations and make good decisions.

Relying on Fast Food

With our busy lifestyles, we often don't have time to cook so we rely on fast food for our meals. Ouch! This can be fatal to weight loss success. Because choices are so limited and we're tired and hurried we tend to gorge ourselves with unhealthy, high-calorie fast foods. It becomes our reward and our release from a hectic day. We use busy lifestyles as an excuse for not eating right.

We behave as if fast food is our only option. Is it? Let's say you just got home from work and you have to rush out the door because your kids have a soccer game. Why not grab a peanut butter sandwich and a banana instead of eating a Big Mac and fries at McDonald's? You think you don't have time to make a quick dinner to go. But do you?

How much time do you spend waiting in busy drive-thru lines, especially at dinnertime? You're more likely to save time by fixing something at home and I guarantee you will feel better for it.

If your excuse is that you go right from work to other activities, how about stopping at a full-service convenience store instead. We have "Wawa" convenience stores where we live. This place is great. It's a mini-grocery store with a full deli. They'll make you any kind of sandwich. They serve fresh soup and always have yogurts, fresh fruit and salads. You can always find a healthier, lower-calorie alternative in the same amount of time as you can get high-calorie junk at the fast food chain.

Fast food joints do offer some healthier choices (although limited and pretty boring). You can get by with a reasonable amount of calories if you make the right choices. Beware of their healthier options. Alternative "healthy" sandwiches or salads made with iceberg lettuce (nearly void of nutritional value) and full-fat dressing along with cheese, croutons and whatever else they use to provide taste can be more calories than a regular hamburger and small fries.

Most fast food places provide nutritional content brochures. Check them out so you can make an educated choice.

Saving Time and Money

Years ago, people ate breakfast at home and brought their lunch to work. Nowadays, we grab a donut, Egg McMuffin or bagel and cream cheese and buy our lunch. I did this for a year when I worked in the city. Not only was I heavier then, but when my husband and I went on a budget, we realized that, between the two of us, we spent over $300 a month buying food at work. When we started eating from home and bringing our lunch more often we saved $200 a month! That was a new car payment in those days! Not only that but we both lost a few pounds without even trying!

We used to have convenience foods a lot when I forgot to defrost something. So many times I would end up waiting at a pizza place for 25 minutes for my order and by the time I got home the pizza was cold and I was more stressed out. While we still do this on occasion, most of the time we opt to eat at home. We can fix a sandwich and a bowl of soup far faster, with much less stress. And again, we save money, too!

Don't Eat on the Run

The other day I saw a guy in his car with a Big Mac in one hand while driving his car with the other. He's eating a 650-calorie sandwich, most likely with a 500-calorie bag of fries at his side and his eating "pleasure" is over before he gets to the next intersection. What a waste of calories!

If you can't set aside enough time in a day to stop what you are doing and eat then you've got to do something to slow down the pace of your lifestyle. If I'm too busy to have a meal, I try to graze a little until I have the time to enjoy a meal. I try not to ever "woof" down a high-calorie meal. It's a waste of calories. Calories I could enjoy when I have more time.

Be Aware of What You Eat

The simple message is to *always be aware of what you eat.* Get into the habit of knowing what, how and why you are eating. Awareness is a great step to avoiding denial. Pay attention to everything you put into your mouth, whether it's eating the leftovers on your kid's plate or grabbing fun size candy bars while running out the door. If you are guilty of these things, then fess up and at least admit to them.

Every time you go to put something in your mouth, ask yourself if you really want it. What am I eating it for? Is it better off in the garbage than in my mouth? Will it spoil my next meal? How am I eating? Am I gobbling my food? Am I eating on the run? Why am I eating, if I'm not even hungry?

Eat only what you want. How much food do you eat in a day that you really don't even want? Enjoy everything you eat and if you aren't enjoying it, don't eat it. Find something worth eating.

Be aware of the quantities. If you are snacking on cookies or chips, take a serving. Know the calorie count of each serving. If you want more you can always go back and get more, but at least you become aware of the amount you are eating.

The problem with learning how to listen to your body is that some of us really don't know how to identify what our body wants or needs. We have been brainwashed by diet books, marketing hype and even news media "exposés." The reality is many of us don't have a clue about food. We're gobbling up misinformation and resisting helpful information. The more educated you are, the better consumer (of food) you'll be. The more you know about your body and what it wants and needs the better you will feel. The more you can recognize and control your bad habits, the more successful you will be.

And if all else fails, try listening to your grandma. Do you remember those rules?

Let's refresh your memory.

- Eat your vegetables
- You can't have dessert until you finish your supper (i.e., eat your vegetables before your cookies)
- You'll spoil your dinner
- Don't talk with your mouth full
- If you eat too much you'll have a belly ache
- Don't leave the house without breakfast
- Turn off the TV
- Go outside and play!
- Go work up an appetite

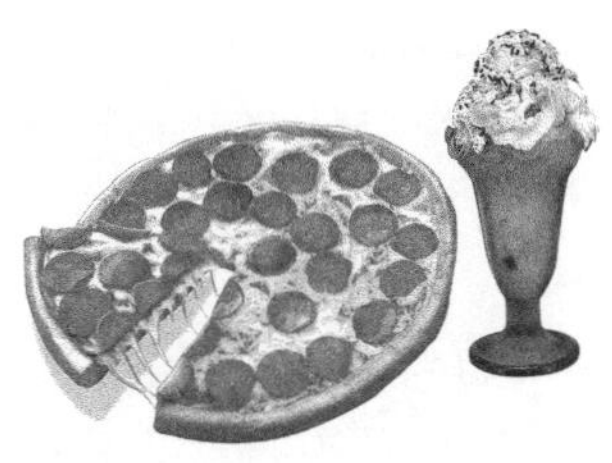

PART III
A New Way of Behaving
The NEW You

If you are mentally ready for change and are willing to practice your listening skills then it's time to work on the NEW You.

- **N**utrition
- **E**xercise
- **W**eight Training

The NEW You formula is guaranteed to make tremendous changes in your life. If your lifestyle consists of good nutrition, regular exercise and weight (resistance) training, you will look better, feel better and be healthier.

The NEW You Diet! The revolutionary, doctor-approved, guaranteed and effective way of losing weight!! Go from this, to this! Doctor-tested, mother-approved! Feel your best, look your best! Eat all the foods you want! Yes, you can even eat pizza and ice cream!

Of course, this is a parody on all the popular diets. But by steering your lifestyle in this direction, favorable results are guaranteed. It sounds strict and complex, but once you get started, it's pretty easy. Making lifestyle changes does take dedication, a little willpower, a learning process and time. But it's really not hard. Trust me!

The degree to which you incorporate these components into your life determines your results. You can design your own nutrition, exercise and weight training program. You can be as aggressive or passive as you want. Give it a try, keep it up and add to it when you are ready. Just don't quit. Accept this way is the only way to look your best and feel your best. Just keep trying and keep learning and one day you will be healthier, happier and achieve your realistic goals.

Nutrition

Try to eat a well-balanced diet. Look to the food pyramid and once you have had your fruit and veggies, have a cookie if you want. If you are trying to lose weight, cut out a serving or two of carbohydrates and reduce the sweets and fats. For best results learn which foods are proteins, fats and carbohydrates. Learn to read labels.

Exercise

Get off your butt. It doesn't matter what you do, just move it! Do no more than you can handle and up the ante only when you're ready. And if you did a real good job today, have another cookie (but not half the bag).

Weight Training

Alternate or combine weight training with exercise. It doesn't take a lot of time and its rewards are well worth the effort. Building muscle is the most effective way to stimulate your metabolism and reshape your body. Weight training keeps your body young.

Sound boring? Been there and done that? Disappointed? Think you can't do it? Well, too bad. If you want permanent change, The NEW You combination will get you where you want to be. It's the only *proven* way to look and feel your best both inside and out. Millions have been successful and most who have stuck with it have no desire to go back. It's the one method you can use for a lifetime. And you know what? You can do it and, if you give it a chance, you will enjoy it. And if you don't achieve your visual goals, what have you lost? You are now living a healthier lifestyle and you feel better. There is no downside.

I'm not going to give you a precise road map on what to do. I'm not going to provide healthy recipes. I won't tell you how much food you can eat or give you an exercise schedule. There are hundreds of books on those subjects. And what specifically worked for me may not work for you. But I can give you guidance and educate you on the basic fundamentals. I can help get you motivated to succeed in the actual "doing." As I said, failure isn't caused by not having a way to do it. The reason is we don't do it!

I encourage you to learn everything you can about nutrition, exercise and weight training. The more educated you are and the better choices you make, the more successful you'll be.

Most of us are not successful because we never learn anything. Most books tell us what to eat and what not to eat. But many don't ever teach you the fundamentals of food. Food marketers develop foods that they claim are "nutritious" and we believe them because we aren't educated enough to know otherwise. Commercials tell us their gadget is easy to use or burns the most calories, but they don't tell you how to motivate yourself to actually get on the darn thing. Gyms advertise their advanced weight lifting equipment, but provide little education in how to use all the stuff.

So let's start learning and let's start doing to become The NEW You!

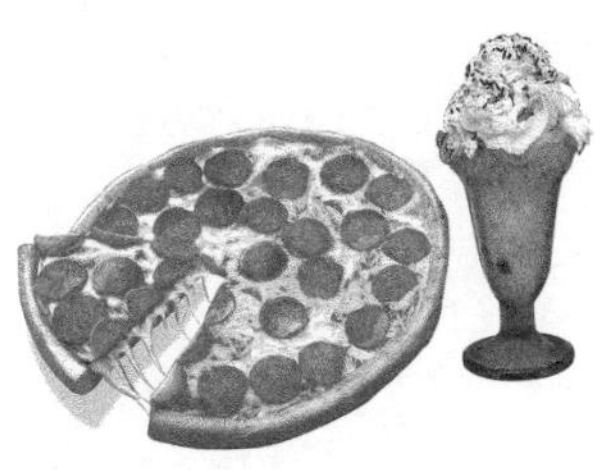

Chapter 14

STEP 7
Nutrition for The NEW You

I've said it before, but I probably need to say it again. The calorie is the primary factor in weight control. Whether you want to lose 5 pounds or 200, if you reduce the amount of calories you feed your body, or increase the calories your body needs, you will lose weight. Your body's caloric needs are largely determined by how much you use it. What kinds of calories you consume determines your overall health and contributes to the ability to keep your caloric intake under control. If you are giving your body the nutrients and calories it needs, it should be satisfied.

In order to design a nutrition plan, you need to learn how to identify the components of food and then determine how much you should eat. To do this we're going to get educated on the components of food:

- Protein
- Fat
- Carbohydrate

You should eat all three in moderation every day. None of the components are "bad" but excessively eating any of them is unhealthy and contributes to weight gain. I'd need an entire book to discuss all the elements of food and nutrition. But there are plenty of books on the subject already. I want to give you a crash course in nutritional reality.

I'm going to give you information you can use. We've heard it all before; sugars are bad; carbohydrates are bad; fats are bad; proteins are bad. We have been misled and misinformed by the diet and food industry and even more disappointing, a few in the medical community. We're not listening to sound practical research but rather the latest news sound bite or infomercial. Let's dissect the truth from fantasy and get educated on the reality of food.

Protein

You should have a serving of protein at every meal. Foods rich in protein are meats, fish, eggs and poultry. Tofu, nuts, soy and legumes are vegetarian sources of protein. The amount of calories per serving of protein does not vary much. The difference in calories from one protein food to another is the fat content in those foods. A gram of protein is four calories. It doesn't matter whether that gram of protein is in beef, chicken, pork, fish, beans, tofu or nuts. Protein is still four calories per gram.

Some foods are good sources of protein (like peanut butter, legumes, cheese) but also contain fat and/or carbohydrates as well.

Calorie for calorie lean protein is the most filling food you can eat. High-protein diets rely on this fact to reduce calorie consumption. However, our bodies seldom crave more than three or four protein servings a day. In fact, excessive amounts of protein can put a strain on your kidneys. The body's natural objection to too much protein can cause nausea, another reason high-protein diets result in temporary weight loss – and a reason why we don't succeed following high-protein diets.

A serving of lean protein is about 18-24 grams or 72-96 calories. There is a small amount of fat in most lean fish and meat proteins. So a lean serving of protein is usually about 100-140 calories. Three servings of lean protein a day are less than 500 calories.

While protein can be very satisfying, our bodies usually don't want more than about one-half gram per pound of body weight per day (a 150-pound person would need about 75 grams of protein). If you have a lot of muscle or are very active, your body may crave a little more.

Is No Meat Best?

There is a misconception that a vegetarian diet is a healthier diet and will help you lose weight. While this may be true in some cases, the absence of meat in a vegetarian diet can cause you to gain weight if other factors are not controlled. Our bodies need protein. Our biggest source of protein is in meat, eggs and fish. Too little protein can inhibit muscle maintenance and growth. If you are vegetarian you shouldn't rely on fats and carbohydrates alone. To satisfy your protein needs, you will need to include tofu, soy, nuts and legumes in your daily diet. Unlike other nutrients, you can't take a protein pill. You can add protein shakes or bars to a vegetarian diet for added protein. However, to me, it's not a palatable way to spend your calories.

While I respect that some of us choose to be vegetarian for moral reasons, choosing to be vegetarian as a way to lose weight is misguided. Some young people become vegetarians because it's in vogue; it's cool. But in many cases, lack of protein contributes to dietary inadequacies in growing bodies.

If you are avoiding protein due to fat, cholesterol or calorie concerns, you shouldn't be. Assuming you are otherwise healthy, if you have a balanced diet, you can have an egg in the morning and lean beef once or twice a week, without adverse results in any category. You should get some of your protein from low-fat, low-cholesterol sources, but you don't need to avoid other protein sources as long as your overall diet is not high in fat.

Keeping Protein Simple

Rather than avoiding certain proteins, just choose to eat them in modified ways. For example, I eat eggs every morning. I eat five eggs: one whole egg and four egg whites – 135 calories with about four grams of fat. Sometimes I throw in leftover vegetables or a sprinkling of cheese. Add two pieces of hearty whole grain bread with a little jelly and you have a wonderful, filling breakfast for about 300 calories. The meal contains about 7 grams of fiber, 24 grams of protein, a little folic acid, calcium and other vital nutrients. Compare this to a bagel with cream cheese, where total calories can soar up to 500 and includes 7 grams of saturated fat, about one gram of fiber and maybe 5 grams of protein.

No time to cook? My husband can throw some egg whites in a pan with cooking spray, put it on a whole-wheat wrap with a little salsa and be on the road in 5 minutes. How much time and money do you spend waiting for your fast food breakfast?

We eat steak about once a week. I typically choose London broil or filet mignon. Too expensive, you say? It's cheaper than a pizza, especially if the meat is on sale at the grocery store. These cuts are lower in fat and moderate in calories. Leaner beef will have less marbling – the white stuff (fat) that runs through the meat. Of course, you should cut off the exterior ends as well.

We also eat a lot of lean pork, chicken, fish and we love ground turkey. I use ground turkey as a replacement for most ground beef, like in meatloaf, pasta sauce, chili and burgers. A well-made turkey burger with a sprinkling of good cheese on a whole-wheat bun is far better tasting than a greasy hamburger with a slab of American cheese. Try it. I guarantee you'll like it and the fat and calorie difference can be as much as 200 calories per sandwich. Not only do you save calories but you also get better nutrition and better taste without sacrificing a thing.

Fat

Consume fat in moderation. If you eat very little fat, you should probably add more fat to your diet. Fat is an essential nutrient. It's satisfying and flavorful. If you are currently eating a high fat diet, you should reduce your fat intake to no more than 30 percent of your daily calories.

The problem is not so much the amount of fat in our diet, but that much of the fat we eat is saturated. Reducing fat is one of the most painless ways to reduce calories. So much of the fat we eat is unnecessary. You can easily remove 200 calories or more from some dishes without altering the taste. In fact, once you discover the true taste of the food that's beneath all the fat, you will realize that the food tastes better when the fat is just an enhancement to the dish.

Many restaurants and processed products rely on "bad" fats for taste. Cheap and most moderately priced restaurants sometimes add outrageous amounts of unnecessary fats (especially saturated fats like butter, cheese and cream) to their foods. Once you modify your fat intake for a while, you will find your taste buds adjust accordingly and you will soon find high-fat foods less desirable.

More expensive restaurants prepare food with less fat and the food is more nutritious. They rely on the flavor of fresh meats, vegetables and spices. Dousing foods in fat does not make them better. Most of us are just used to the taste of fat because we eat so much of it.

I talk with many people looking for low-fat recipes. They'll say, "I want to eat less fat but how do I cook that way?"

Generally, you don't need a new recipe book to modify fats in your cooking. Most recipes can easily be altered. By reducing the oil, butter and cheese, or substituting lower fat milk you can still maintain the flavor of recipes without ruining the result. As long as you know what a fat is, you can reduce it. You don't need to learn how to cook all over again. It does help to learn options to replace fat for added flavor, for example, wine, skim milk, spices or vegetable broth in lieu of some of the fat.

The exception is in baked goods and fried foods. Unlike cooking, baking is a science and measurements and consistency are important. Fried foods are what they are. You "fry" in oil, so if you omit the oil, it's not fried anymore

"Good" Fat, "Bad" Fat

Let's not forget that while all fats contain the same amount of calories (9 calories per gram or about 100 calories per tablespoon), there are different kinds of fats. While I keep saying there are no "good" foods or "bad" foods, I can say there are "good" fats and "bad" fats.

Bad Fats

Saturated fats are those that come mainly from animal sources and certain tropical oils such as coconut and palm. The liver uses saturated fats to manufacture cholesterol. The more saturated fat in your diet, the more cholesterol your liver will produce.

Hydrogenated fats are found in margarines, vegetable shortening and nearly every manufactured processed food. Hydrogenated fat is sometimes labeled as artificially saturated. The oil becomes saturated during processing from a liquid to a solid. As a general rule, if a fat stays solid at room temperature, it's either saturated or hydrogenated.

Judith Shaw, author of *Raising Low-Fat Kids in a High-Fat World*, says these fats are found in almost every processed food in the supermarket from soups to chips, crackers to cookies, pastries to mixes of all kinds including some pasta and rice mixes.

When reviewing how much fat you eat a day, consider how

much of the fat you eat is saturated or hydrogenated. I think you will be shocked at the amount of "bad" fat you actually eat.

The Deceiving Horror Story

While we may be passing up the protein to avoid saturated fats, we most likely are consuming copious amounts of hydrogenated fats in all the processed food we eat. Current nutritional labeling does not require disclosure of hydrogenated fat grams per serving of foods. We see a low percentage of saturated fat and assume the food is okay. You can't decipher how much hydrogenated fat is in the food you are eating so it is difficult to make better choices. For example, if a label shows eight grams of fat, and two grams are saturated and the food contains hydrogenated oil (listed in the ingredients) you have no way of knowing how much of the remaining six grams is due to the hydrogenated oil! It's outrageous! The public is not being fully informed about the ingredients in the food. There is legislation pending to require such labeling, but as for now, it's a guessing game.

Good Fats

On the other hand, some fats might actually lower cholesterol. Monounsaturated fats are the good guys. They are found mostly in olive oil, canola oil, safflower oil and many nuts like almonds, cashews and peanuts. Mono fats appear to reduce blood levels of the LDL's (low density lipoprotein) without affecting HDL's (high density lipoprotein). LDL's are the "bad" guys, HDL's are the "good" guys.

Responding to the importance of monounsaturated fats in our diet, Alice Lichtenstein, Ph.D., professor of nutrition at Tufts University, says, "It's not enough to reduce total calories from fat in our diet. We need to also pay attention to what types of fats we are consuming."

Polyunsaturated fats are somewhere in the middle. Polyunsaturated fats can reduce harmful LDL's, but can also reduce HDL's, the good cholesterol. Some polyunsaturated fats are vegetable, corn, soybean and sunflower seed oil.

The best fat choice is Omega 3-fatty acids that are found in many types of fish, especially salmon. I find it interesting that some of the fat in animal proteins can increase cholesterol while fish fat may help to lower cholesterol.

Dissecting fats from the good and bad can be confusing. As a general rule, you should limit your fat intake to no more 30 percent of total calories per day. Of that, only 10 percent should be from bad fats. However, *reducing bad fats to **any** lower percentage is a good place to start.*

Keeping Fat Simple

If you are confused about everything I just said, I'll try to make it as simple as possible. To control your cholesterol and help maintain or lose weight, you need to eat less processed foods and keep your fat intake to no more than 30 percent of total calories. Most of your diet should come from whole foods – fruits, vegetables, lean protein, whole grains and *"good"* fats. Stay away from processed foods as much as possible. Cook with good oils (like canola or olive oil) at home and reserve your "bad" fat intake for treats you really want to enjoy.

It sounds restrictive, but it's really not. You can work your bad fats into a healthy diet. For example, I try to keep my overall fat intake below the 30 percent maximum. For maintenance, I eat about 1,800 - 2,000 calories per day. If I keep my fat intake to no more than 30 percent of total calories, I can eat up to 60 grams or 540 calories per day in fat. That's a reasonable amount of fat.

I always cook with olive or canola oil. We also have fish once or twice a week. We eat lean meats. I like nuts that contain "good" fat, but I also like my crackers and ice cream. I like cheese, but I use it more as a condiment. I also choose densely flavored cheese like asiago or feta. A little bit goes a long way for flavor. I also have my occasional days with pizza and french fries.

On average, I eat about 20 grams, or 180 calories, of saturated fat a day – about 10 percent of total daily calories. Even if I go over my "bad" fat allowance a little, it can be offset by the good oils I eat. So it's a balance.

If you are eating a lot of fat in your diet, start making better choices. If 50 percent of your calories are from fat and 40 percent of them are from bad fats, it's bad news. Start cutting back on fat, particularly bad fat, wherever you can. Continue to cut back but don't make the goal overwhelming. You can substitute monounsaturated fats for saturated fats without changing the taste. *Every little bit helps.* Do it for your (and your family's) health. Just start trying and keep it up. Soon you will find your palate will adapt to the changes and you can gradually cut more fat (especially bad fat) out of your diet. You won't miss a thing.

Carbohydrates

Unless your meals come out of a Jack Daniels bottle, any food you eat that is not a fat or protein is a carbohydrate. To say carbohydrates are evil is absolutely ridiculous. Living on mostly fat and protein is evil! You should eat carbohydrates in moderation depending on your activity level. Carbohydrates give us energy to do the active things we should be doing. The amount of carbs you consume relative to your fat and protein intake depends on your activity level and how fast your motor (your metabolism) is running.

If you sit at a desk all day, then hang out on the Internet or "veg" in front of the TV, then your body doesn't need a lot of carbohydrates. But then again, it doesn't need a lot of calories either.

For nutrition, the type of carbohydrate you eat can make the difference for weight control and health. All vegetables and fruits are carbohydrates, but so is table sugar and flour.

Since carbohydrates encompass so many of the foods we eat, both densely and minimally nutritious, there is much confusion over the food group. People are misled and misinformed. The diet industry has perpetuated the problem by generalizing the value of carbohydrates. We are listening to the hype du jour without looking for validation and ignoring the vast majority of nutrition experts.

Knowing the Difference

We all know fruits, vegetables and whole grains are the best carbohydrate choices. For all other carbohydrate choices, look for fiber and protein content. The more fiber and protein, the less the food has been processed and the healthier it is. A piece of whole grain bread may contain five grams of protein and five grams of fiber. A piece of white bread, on the other hand may contain only one gram of protein and near zero in fiber. High-fiber carbohydrates digest slowly in your system, prevent insulin spikes and give you sustained energy. Calorie for calorie, fiber-rich foods will keep you satisfied longer, are better for you and actually taste better.

The Next Dietary Fears

There has been a lot of talk recently about the glycemic index of carbohydrates. The glycemic index ranks foods according to how they affect our blood sugar levels. The index measures how much your blood sugar increases after eating a particular food and can be particularly important for diabetics.

Twenty years ago, scientists thought "sugar" only applied to simple sugars. Simple sugars are sometimes referred to as "empty" calories, meaning that the food provides little nutritional value. Now, we find that other carbohydrates are "simple" sugars and can raise blood sugars nearly as high as table sugar. The most common type of high glycemic foods is white flour. There are even a few fruits and vegetables such as carrots and watermelon that have high glycemic levels.

I haven't been able to find research that determines how much is too much when it comes to high-glycemic foods. I'm not sure if a specific number is even known at this time. You can find glycemic tables on dozens of web sites, but rather than get bogged down with yet another list of confusing food "no-no's," I prefer to use the philosophy that if you get most of your calories from lean protein, moderate consumptions of good fats and whole food carbohydrates like fruits, vegetables and whole grains, your diet won't consist of too many high-glycemic foods anyway.

The problem is not that high-glycemic foods are necessarily bad for you. The greater problem is that more and more of today's foods are highly processed and therefore, are likely to be high-glycemic. And because we're eating more and more processed foods, we're likely to be eating more high-glycemic foods.

Eating Carbohydrates Sensibly

With misinformed thinking, we believe we have to restrict most carbohydrates, especially carbs that aren't fruits or vegetables. Like fat, you don't have to give them up, just consume them in moderation. Work them into a nutritionally balanced diet.

To figure out how you are going to moderate calories and carbohydrates you need to pick and choose carbohydrates wisely. My main choices for carbohydrates are vegetables and whole grains. While I try to have at least two fruit choices a day, I don't eat a lot of fruit, unless it's in season. While fruit contains fiber and vitamins, it also can be fairly caloric. I consume a lot of fresh vegetables, particularly large quantities of nutritious options, nearly every night for dinner – broccoli, beans and asparagus, along with a dark green salad. As a general rule, the darker the vegetable, the more nutritious. Iceberg lettuce, for example, has very little nutritional value yet many uninformed people will rely on iceberg lettuce topped with high-fat dressing as their main source of nutrition.

I crave a little fruit mid-morning, but at night I want my ice cream or chocolate treat. If I consume a lot of fruit, I won't have reserved calories to enjoy my treat.

I'm sure I touched a few nerves with that preference so let me clarify. It would be *better* if I didn't do this, but I like my ice cream. I like my M&M's. If I eat more fruit and still crave the M&M's, I'm probably going to have the fruit *and* the M&M's. In the end I'm going to consume more calories. I generally eat very healthy foods, so if I'd rather have a cookie than an apple, I think I can and not beat myself up about it.

I also moderate calories by only choosing the less nutritious carbohydrates I truly want. For example, I want my after dinner treat and I also like snack crackers or pretzels with my lunch. To balance my calories and carbohydrate consumption, I usually pass up the dinner starch because, for me, it's not that important.

The Evils of Nutritional Labeling

As I said, one of the biggest problems with our diets today is the average person is getting most of their calories from fat and highly processed foods that contain very little nutrients. Remember the more processed the food, the fewer nutrients are in them. Food producers are now adding some unnatural nutrients back into processed foods in an effort to make them "healthier," a process often referred as "enriching" the food.

Although the addition of vitamins and minerals to processed foods technically makes them somewhat healthier for you, it discourages people from eating unprocessed, naturally healthy foods. This growing trend is a pet peeve of mine. We refuse to eat healthy foods so we rely on processed food with added vitamins as our solution to better eating. It's a downward spiral and I think it is outrageous. Wake up and think about what we are doing! We are adding a vitamin pill to our sugar and fat products all in the name of better health.

Seeing the niche in food labeling, marketers of food products are using the term "healthier" to lure uneducated, yet well-intended consumers to buy their product. What's worse, the main ingredients in some of these so-called "nutritious" products include hydrogenated oils and another growing menace, high fructose corn syrup. High fructose corn syrup has been shown to raise triglyceride levels, which can increase the risk of heart disease. So now you have a nutritionally void food containing the worst kind of fat and sugars with claims that they are healthy!

If you are eating these foods just because they contain vitamins and minerals you may want to save the calories and take a vitamin pill instead. Focus more on eating "real" food rather than nutritionally "enriched" processed foods. The entire marketing craze is moving us further away from a healthy diet and discouraging us from eating naturally nutritious foods. Here are a few misconceptions many of us are buying into:

Sports Drinks and Juices

The primary ingredient in most sports drinks and juices is sugar, usually high fructose corn syrup. Juices contain lots of sugar, and that means plenty of calories. Unless their body needs refueling, most exercisers need neither one.

Sports drinks are good for someone who is exercising intensely for over an hour especially in the heat where you need fast refueling and hydration. For most of us who are playing an hour of doubles tennis or doing a half hour on the stair stepper, water is all you need. Moreover, these drinks add calories, reducing the benefits of your workout. And they are expensive!

Most fruit drinks contain a minimal amount of real fruit juice and even the 100 percent juice should be consumed in moderation. Why? They are very high in calories, almost as high as some brands of soda. One hundred percent juice does contain some vitamin benefits and I'm not saying you should eliminate your morning orange juice. What I am saying is that excessive amounts do not benefit your diet and just lead to excessive calorie consumption.

Children are often big juice drink consumers. Excessive amounts of sugar, particularly high fructose corn syrup, can cause diarrhea and hyperactivity in sugar sensitive children and can add to weight gain. A recent study at Boston Children's Hospital found that drinking one soft drink *or* sweetened fruit juice a day gives a kid a 60 percent greater chance of becoming obese.

Most kids aren't allowed to bring candy to school in their lunches. Yet, most children bring in so-called "juice" drinks: Hi-C, Hawaiian Punch, and Capri-Sun, just to name a few. Other than a little vitamin C, the ingredients in these juices are sugar, flavoring and water. I never understood the wisdom of allowing juice drinks, but banning Skittles.

I'm not encouraging schools to allow candy at school, but to allow one and not the other is ridiculous. I can't tell you how many times a mother will say "no" to her kids' desire for soda and then give them a Hi-C instead. I prefer my son drink a caffeine-free Diet Pepsi instead of fruit juice. I see people give me the "you're-a-bad-mother" look for allowing soda, especially diet soda, over fruit juice. I'm not saying one is better than the other, but I'm not clear on the argument that juice drinks are "good" while soda is "bad." All I know is water is better.

The best sports drink is water. Our bodies need a lot of water (at least 8 glasses a day) to maintain good health. The more water, the better. Many of us, especially children, are not getting enough water in our diet and are relying on sugared water as our main source of hydration.

Bottled water is a good way to encourage more water consumption. While it may seem silly to buy water, the convenience factor makes water consumption easier. I grab a water bottle for the car ride when I do errands. It doesn't spill and you can even put it in your purse. It also helps ward off hunger pains.

It's especially great for children. Kids like packaging. A water bottle is "cool." My kids like water bottles but snub their nose at a glass of water.

Energy Bars/Drinks

Energy bars and drinks offer "balanced nutrition" on the run. It's okay as a last resort for busy people trying to stick with a healthier diet. I know my college son and his roommates like to keep them on hand when running back and forth to class when the only thing in the fridge is a lone beer and fuzzy Chinese food.

The misconception of an energy bar is it provides some kind of enhancement or ability to get you fit or to lose weight. Most energy bars contain 200-300 calories. While they may contain some protein, vitamins and minerals and are low in fat, most contain sugar, additives, preservatives and hydrogenated oils, and most contain little fiber. A can of Slim Fast has a whopping 35 grams of sugar – 64 percent of total calories. The next time you're at the grocery store, pick up a few different meal replacement bars and drinks and look at the actual food ingredients, not just the vitamin/mineral content. Nutrition and caloric content vary a lot between brands. Read the labels before you decide.

While there is nothing wrong with eating an "energy" bar or drink, I don't find any of them appetizing and the more "nutritional" the energy bar claims to be, the worst it tastes, especially the high protein bars. Either way, it's still calories. If you are eating energy bars in addition to your diet, you're just adding more calories.

The PBJ – Nature's Energy Bar

My favorite energy bar is a peanut butter and jelly sandwich. If it's on Roman Meal 12-grain bread with one tablespoon of peanut butter and a bit of jelly, the nutritional value is about 300 calories - 10 grams of protein, 7 grams of fiber and about 8 grams of fat (mostly good fat). Total fat equals about 24 percent of calories.

So, if you are eating an energy bar to replace a peanut butter sandwich, the latter tastes much better and is more satisfying. Don't sacrifice real food with a meal replacement bar unless you have no other nutritional food option or prefer the taste (although I can't imagine that).

"Healthy" Snack Bars

Many of the nutritional snack alternatives are not much better than a candy bar. If you look at the nutritional ingredients, most are simply processed carbohydrates with a few added vitamins. They contain very little nutritional benefits and simply add calories to your diet. Not that it's wrong, but it needs to be identified for what it is.

Don't be fooled into thinking that a Nutri-Grain cereal bar is significantly healthier for you than a half a candy bar. While they may have less fat, they can contain as much sugar, especially the low-fat ones. The snack industry has recently started marketing a new granola bar that contains popular candy bar products in them. Basically it's a candy bar mixed with a little granola. "Look Mom, buy our snack bars, they've got nutritious granola in them!" How ridiculous. My advice is to hop on the Internet and learn how to make your own granola bars. They're cheap, easy to make and more nutritious.

Keep an eagle eye on the nutritional labels too. They can be deceiving. A granola bar, for example, contains about 10 grams of sugar while a candy bar may contain 20 grams. At first glance, it appears that the candy bar has more sugar. However, what most of us don't realize is the granola bar is half the calories (and often, half the size) of the candy bar. While a chocolate bar will contain more fat, calorie for calorie, the bar has just as much sugar. So if you are looking for something sweet decide whether you would rather have a dry granola bar (about 130 calories) or two Ghirardelli chocolate squares (about 140 calories). I know which one I would rather have.

We think a Nutri-Grain bar is a healthy quick breakfast for our kids but a Pop Tart isn't. In reality, the Pop Tart has about the same nutritional value and food component distribution as the Nutri-Grain bar. The only significant difference is that a Pop Tart has 50 more calories.

"Healthy" sounding snack bars give parents peace of mind when analyzing the visual nutritional content of their kid's lunch box. If the product says "granola," "nutri" or "healthy" parents will buy it. The words make the product seem healthy. We hand it out guilt free.

The bottom line is if you want a processed granola bar, have one. But if you want something nutritious, have an apple. If you want a treat, don't settle for the dry "healthy" bar. You'll be more satisfied with the candy bar. Just make sure the candy bar is a small part of an otherwise healthy diet.

Fibbing: The "Light, Natural, Healthy" Way

You have to be careful of misleading labels. Don't assume that because the label reads "light," "natural" or "healthy" it is a diet or healthy food.

The best way to make a healthier choice is to read the nutritional and ingredient label. For general nutrition, I look for foods that contain around 30 percent or less in fat and contain fiber and/or protein. I read the ingredients and compare calories to portions. Most savvy food labelers try to keep snack food's "serving" size at about 150-200 calories. If the calories in a product are higher, they just reduce the quantity per serving so the food doesn't look so fattening. If a food is high in carbohydrates and contains very little protein or fiber, the carbs are probably processed carbohydrates, which provides necessary fuel but little nutrition.

Calorie for calorie (or gram for gram), a slice of white bread will leave you less satisfied than a slice of whole wheat bread. I don't pay much attention to foods that have added vitamins and minerals unless the food itself is the source of the nutrition. I can take a vitamin pill as easily as ingesting a sugared cereal laced with added vitamins. "Light" doesn't mean low calorie, just as "natural" doesn't necessarily mean unprocessed. I've never seen a guideline for using the word "healthy." It's just a word. Low fat doesn't mean low calorie and low fat doesn't necessarily mean better for you.

What's better for you, too much sugar or too much fat? Too much of either one isn't good. While I look for good nutritious foods as part of a healthy diet, I don't look for nutrition when having a treat. I'd rather have a good chocolate bar than a Nutri-Grain bar.

Making Wiser Choices

If you are relying on "healthy" versions of processed foods as a solution to your poor eating habits, you are not solving your problem. Get most of your calories from whole foods. The philosophy of purchasing your foods from the perimeter of a grocery store is a great recommendation. Meats (protein), vegetables and dairy are typically on the outside walls of a grocery store while processed products – canned goods, cereals, candy, cookies, chips, frozen foods, etc., are in the middle.

Buy most of your foods on the perimeter and then choose your "treats" carefully from the middle. Decide what "treats" you want and don't buy what you really don't want. Don't buy the large box of cookies because they are cheap and convenient and don't buy the "fat-free" kind simply because of the label. Hold out for the Nestle Toll House cookies and bake them on a Saturday after you worked in the yard for a couple of hours.

Don't judge a food by its packaging. If you learn the value of food you can be a better food consumer and you won't be misled by shadowy marketing and packaging gimmicks. Read the side of the box (the nutrition and ingredients label), not the front. Pay special attention to weight and serving size.

But What and How Much Should I Eat?

I can't tell you how much you should eat. If you can admit to what you really eat, you should find your answer. Eat fewer calories than you do now. Apply basic nutrition principles and daily caloric recommendations if you need guidance. Learn about the quality of foods. You should strive to make healthy choices first for your health. However, you don't need to eat only healthy foods to be healthy or to lose weight. Don't get too caught up in the "good" food, "bad" food theories. Confusion over what to eat discourages people from trying. It becomes too complicated, restrictive and misleading. If you listen to your body, it will tell you what it wants and how much. It will crave good nutrition and it will tell you when it's full and it doesn't mind a french fry or cookie once in a while either.

Journal Keeping

If you need assistance in determining where you need to change your diet, keep a food journal. A journal determines your starting point – a baseline. Once you determine what you eat now, you can decide how you are going to moderate calories and add healthier foods to your diet. It tells you where you are now so you can move in a better, healthier direction.

Journal keeping can also help you identify other negative lifestyle behaviors like exercise frequency and bad habits. While journal keeping can guide you through the lifestyle change process, the overall objective is to help you overcome your obstacles so you don't need to keep a journal anymore

Nutritional labeling on food products and at fast food restaurants will help you determine your baseline. I suggest you purchase a good calorie/nutrient reference paperback. They are usually available at any drug store.

Keep a journal for one week. Don't adjust your diet, be as precise as possible and don't cheat! It's going to be hard to admit that you had 10 cookies last night, not 3; or four servings of pasta, not one. Remember, it doesn't work if you are in denial and not being honest with yourself. If you go through this process and either cheat or eat less or healthier because you want your journal to look good, you aren't being honest and your results will be skewed.

Once you determine how much you are eating and moving now (awareness alone can cause you to eat less and move more) you can plan ways to cut back on your food consumption. You should try to cut back your food consumption by no more than 20 percent. For example, if you average 2,250 calories a day, try to cut your calories by 450 a day. But remember, if you only cut your calories by 100 one day, don't consider it a failure. Every bit helps. And if you eat more than normal (for you) one day, put it behind you. Tomorrow is another day.

You should also analyze what types of food you are eating. Are you getting at least five servings of fruits or vegetables a day? How about calcium and protein? How many processed foods do you eat in a week? Take a good look at what you eat each day and find ways to modify your diet so that you eat healthier and consume fewer calories without feeling like you are "on a diet."

You Don't Know What You're Missing

Changing our food preferences may seem impossible. We assume that we would never want to eat steamed vegetables rather than fried foods. We feel eating healthy is a sacrifice.

Ten years ago I didn't believe it either. Now that I appreciate lower fat, nutritionally dense foods, I enjoy food so much more. I don't eat the way I do now because I feel I have to – I prefer it. I believe if you give yourself a chance to enjoy healthier foods, you will too.

Slowly change your palate to tame your desire for the taste of excessive amounts of fat or sugar. Experiment with new flavors. Pay attention to how the food really tastes, not just how you think it tastes. Move towards a healthier diet. Drastically changing the way you eat is difficult but slow changes, over time, can produce unbelievable results.

Home Alone III

Recently, I was alone for two days. The kids were at Grandma's and my husband was out of town. Ten years ago, an occasion to eat dinner alone would have meant a junk food fest with maybe a Whopper and onion rings. I probably would have stopped by the bakery for a special "treat" because I was alone and I didn't have to acknowledge, justify or share my food with anyone.

Today, it's a different story. While I still thought it was kind of fun to be by myself and eat and do whatever I wanted, the first day I had a leftover turkey burger with pretzels and ice cream. I spent the evening writing this book and playing games of "Free Cell" on the computer to my heart's content.

The second day I took the afternoon off and played golf. On the way home, I stopped at a local gourmet shop and picked up a prepared chicken breast topped with roasted peppers and pesto sauce. I sautéed some asparagus spears and made a salad of spinach, tomatoes and sunflower seeds topped off with light balsamic walnut dressing. I added a whole grain roll and I completed the delicious ensemble with a glass of Sauvignon Blanc. I put on a little music and sat, by myself, enjoying every moment. I was in heaven.

The stop at the gourmet store took 5 minutes and it took 10 minutes to prepare my meal. In both situations, 10 years ago and today, I mentally experienced the same splurge of food – having exactly what I wanted. The difference is that today I value food in a different way.

Even when I was a healthy eater but still obsessing, I would have been tempted to do the "drive-thru" because I thought the junk food was what I really wanted. Eating healthy foods was enjoyable, but I mentally labeled it a sacrifice. Now I'm not tempted by the junk food because I don't want it or even like it.

I didn't become a healthy eater overnight. It was a gradual change. I made small changes and it progressed to bigger changes. I learned the nutritional value of food along the way. I discovered new tastes and lost the desire for old ones. Unfortunately, along the way I got caught up in the mental obsession that eating moderately and healthy was some kind of sacrifice. Once I recognized that my eating habits were a natural desire, not a sacrifice, I could allow all the fun foods to come back into my life and enjoy them again without guilt or fear.

But How Much Can I Eat?

You're probably still waiting for me to tell you what to eat.

Sorry, I'm not going to tell you. I can tell you to eat until you are satisfied – not until you're stuffed. Try to recognize the feeling of being satisfied by eating slower, paying attention to and enjoying your food. Think about whether you really want more food. Give your body a chance to tell you. Make healthier choices in the foods you eat. Consider eating healthier a reward, not a punishment. Learn the nutritional value of foods. Make learning about food values a hobby. Get educated. Control bad habits that encourage overeating.

The key is consistency. Do this for the rest of your life. You don't have to be good every day to be successful but don't quit. If you continuously do this, one day you will find yourself preferring to pass up the fries and going for the broccoli instead. As a general guideline remember the following:

- Use the food pyramid as your guide
- Learn the value of foods
- Fruits, vegetables, lean protein and whole grains should be your dietary mainstay – work towards accomplishing this, but you don't have to do it all at once.
- Don't rely on cleverly marketed, processed foods as your source of nutrition
- Identify where you are now. Figure out how many calories you honestly eat a day and how nutritious is your diet. Start from there and make small changes. Adapt, and progress.

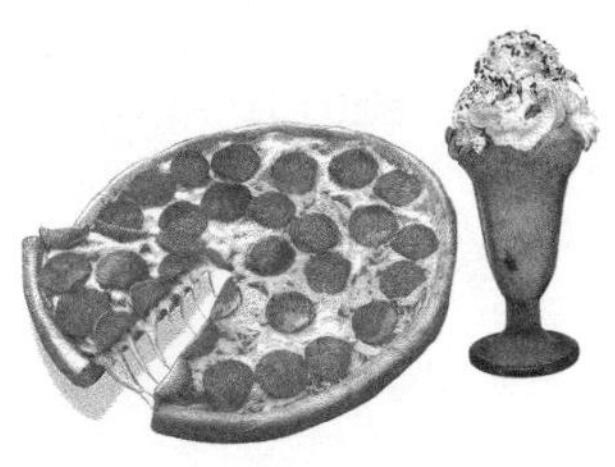

Chapter 15

STEP 8
Exercise for The NEW You

Exercise is the second all-important component to the NEW You. Our bodies need regular exercise in order to be healthy and getting it shouldn't be a necessity only when we want to lose weight. Lack of exercise can be more of a factor in obesity and related illnesses than our diet.

If you get enough exercise every day, you will burn more calories, but more importantly, you feel better and your perception of food changes. You start to experience the "feel good" advantage of exercise and it spills over into your eating habits and lifestyle. Regular exercise is uplifting to the spirit and can reduce emotional eating and mild depression.

If I go two days without a dose of exercise, my good eating habits suffer. I've had times when I've had a fork in my hand with the full intention of picking away at the rest of the peach pie until it was gone. In a split second of recognizing just how much worse I would feel if I did it, I took a walk instead. When I returned, not only did I feel better, I didn't want the pie anymore.

If you haven't discovered the joy of exercising, you probably consider it a bad word like "diet." That's unfortunate. Such preconceived thoughts are sabotaging the fact that exercise can be fun – even more fun than food. When you exercise, food becomes more enjoyable and more fun.

Like eating, in order to make exercise a part of your lifestyle, you have to transition your attitudes about exercise from "I have to" to "I want to." It's easier said than done. But once you know how to get started, learn to listen to your body's signals, not your mind, and experience the joy you will find exercise to be a fun part of your life.

A Fun Day

A perfect day for me would be to walk 18 holes of golf and then have a beer and a turkey club sandwich followed by some kind of ice cream treat. Beer never tastes better and food is great, no matter what it is!

After a day like that I can eat what I want and enjoy every morsel, guilt free, because I earned it. Even if I eat a lot of calories, my body doesn't feel bloated or full. The food tastes so much better than if I got off the couch and ate half as much. My body is screaming for food. Carbs, fat, anything and my body appreciates it.

The Good Old Days

Years ago, we had to move. Today, moving is optional. We don't have to move anymore so we don't. Our environment is so different. Exercise used to be an integral part of our daily life. Now it's one more item on our "to do" list and it usually makes its way to the bottom. Just think about how we lived years ago. Think about all the people who lived off the land: up at dawn to tend the animals, plant or harvest crops all day. No wonder they could eat sausages and flapjacks for breakfast and not even think about getting on a treadmill!

Even a few generations ago, people often lived in towns where you would walk to the corner market, not drive to the major superstore. Television was a luxury and kids' programming was limited to Saturday morning cartoons and a Disney movie on Sunday nights. Not only that but we had to actually get off the couch to change the channel. Video games and computers were pipedreams and your mother did all the housework (in pearls perhaps?).

I remember as a kid, if I wanted to go to a friend's house two miles away, my mom wouldn't take me, I had to walk! Your dad didn't have lawn service, cleaning people were for the rich, your mom hung the laundry on the clothesline on nice days and she ironed your dad's shirts. Terms like "cardio" or "aerobic" were foreign to most of us and few people had a membership to a gym.

If You Like to Eat, You Have to Move

Then times changed. We stopped moving so we started to gain weight. We stopped making meals from scratch. Instead we started to rely on high-fat, fast food. We started eating too much, became fatter, and accordingly, moved our bodies even less. Now we suffer from the consequences.

Because sedentary lifestyles don't keep us moving, we have to schedule our movement. Now we have to "exercise." But exercise doesn't have to mean running three miles or sweating at a high intensity for 45 minutes on a cardio machine. To be cardiovascular healthy you should exercise aerobically for 20 minutes at least three times per week. Aerobically doesn't mean to exhaustion. To develop healthy cardio respiratory systems you simply need to elevate your heart rate about 52 more beats per minute than at rest. It really isn't that hard. A brisk walk will do it.

However, if you just do the minimum, you only burn about 500 calories per week, so don't expect to do the minimum and lose 2 pounds a week. While this may be discouraging, if you continue to do at least the minimum you should lose a pound about every four to six weeks (assuming calories remain the same). So just by doing the minimum, you could theoretically lose about 6 pounds in a year.

Many of us are unsuccessful because we don't see results fast enough. We try to lose 10 pounds by making ourselves miserable trying to do too much, too soon. Then we give up. This is too hard! We need to ease into a new lifestyle and find joy in it.

Just Move More

While there is nothing wrong with exercising at high intensity, most of us are resistant to it, and some of us are physically unable to do it.

But you can burn a lot of calories just by moving more throughout the day or just increasing the intensity at which you move. Many of us are not just resistant to exercise – we are resistant to moving!

On a beautiful day, I watch people blocking traffic waiting for a parking space for up to 5 minutes when there are other spaces available 25 steps more distant. Do you realize I am parked and in the store before they even get into that space? They wasted time (something everyone says they don't have) and they exerted fewer calories than I did.

We avoid movement. If we could just make a small effort to move more than we have to, the difference could be pounds lost over the course of a year.

Many of us move slowly. Watch yourself move. Do you shuffle or do you stride? How about the stairs? Do you run or walk up, stair by stair? How quickly do you get out of the car and into a store?

If you make choices that involve more movement throughout the day, you could easily work off an equivalent of 20 minutes walking on the treadmill. Just putting a little "spring" in your step can help a lot.

Pump Up the Volume

One of the best "move" motivators is music. No matter what you do – cardio machine, walking or housecleaning – you will perform better with music.

Better yet, put on a good tune and dance in your living room. You don't have to go anywhere, you don't need any equipment and everyone can do it in his or her own "unique" way. It may sound ridiculous, but I guarantee you it's easy, fun and when you're done, you'll be smiling. My mom used to dance around the house for 10 minutes a day. She called it her "onesies, twosies."

Sometimes We Surprise Ourselves

One day last month, I dropped off my car at the auto body shop a few miles from my home. I thought I didn't need the car that day but then realized I had to pick up my son from his after school activity. My husband was in a meeting and my oldest son wasn't answering his cell phone. I started to panic. I had about an hour before I had to pick him up. My neighbors weren't home and I was furious that my oldest son wasn't there when I needed him.

Then I had a brainstorm. It was a brisk, 40-degree sunny day, and since the dog hadn't been for a walk in several days I bundled up and started walking. Within 5 minutes I stopped being mad at my son (after all he couldn't know), and I felt invigorated and warm.

A few minutes later, my cell phone rang and it was my son. He apologized and said he'd come pick me up. Happily, I told him "That's okay, I think I'll walk!" I had a wonderful walk with the dog and picked up my car in plenty of time to get my other son.

Some people seem surprised I did this. To me, it made more sense to walk three miles with a specific purpose than to walk the same distance on a treadmill and not even go anywhere!

For many people my solution would not even be an option. Walking three miles to get a car! We think we can't do it because it sounds like exercise and you have to be an "exercise" person to do it. In reality, most people could easily walk three miles and it's even easier if you are doing it for a purpose.

What Are You Listening To?

"I'm too tired" is a typical excuse for not exercising. But what is tired? If you spent six hours doing yard work, or work as a waitperson, landscaper or other labor-intensive job, you really might be tired.

But if you haven't used your body all day, your mind, not your body, is tired. Like our food behavior, we tend to listen to our mind, not our body. Since we're mentally tired after work we think our bodies are tired. The opposite is true.

If you have been at a desk all day, your body wants to get up, stretch and move around. If you come home, eat and then lie on the couch watching TV, surfing the Net or reading a book, you're not in touch with your body's needs. What you need to do is stop thinking and get moving!

Easier Said Than Done

If your thoughts are steering you in the direction of the comfy couch, the thought of exercising is grueling. I know. I feel the same way sometimes – actually most of the time. Don't think because I have been an avid exerciser for years I don't have a problem getting motivated. What keeps me committed is the realization that if I don't get regular exercise, I'm not going to be that happy, energetic person who really enjoys life. It's like a wonder drug. My whole attitude on life can change in 20 minutes.

Once you get into the habit of getting regular exercise, you will appreciate the great feeling afterwards and the thought of not doing it overrides the negative initial feelings of doing it. The

"I'll-do-it-tomorrow" attitude diminishes when you recognize the negative outcome of that decision. The "decision" is not about the total number of calories you are going to burn, but deciding how you want to feel going forward.

Like eating, getting the negative mental thoughts out of the way so you can listen to your body is not easy. The mind is more powerful, so you have to trick it.

Listen to Your Body's Signals

Is Your Body Screaming to Move?

Are you restless? Are you feeling down? Are you irritable? Do you have trouble sleeping at night? Are you always feeling tired? Are you stiff when you get up off the couch? Do you move slowly? Are you always cold and wanting to curl up with a blanket? Typically, we use these symptoms as an excuse not to exercise.

Get out of denial. You know darn well exercise is only going to make your symptoms better. So ask yourself, why wouldn't I try to do something about it! It's like not taking your medicine to cure your illness. Many of us don't take how we feel seriously. We don't respond until our life is at stake. Some of the healthiest people are those who had life-threatening heart attacks early in life. It shouldn't take a wake up call like that to get you moving!

Think About How You Will Feel Afterward

Focus not on how you feel getting started, but how you will feel when you are done – relaxed, proud of yourself and in a better mood. As I've said before, I've never known of anyone who said, "Gee, I wish I didn't exercise."

Think About Your Health

We place too much emphasis on the visual aspect of exercise and not our well-being. Forget about losing 10 pounds. Regular exercise should be as important to you as brushing your teeth or getting a mammogram. I've said this before and it's pretty depressing, but if you are an extremely overweight, inactive person, you're committing slow-motion suicide. The end result will likely be a premature death.

According to the *Journal of Applied Physiology*, just being inactive contributes to at least 17 chronic diseases and is responsible for 25,000 deaths in the U.S. each year. More people die from lack of exercise than from alcohol, firearms, illicit drugs and motor vehicle accidents combined.

Our bodies are meant to move. We stop moving and our bodies start shutting down. The more we move, the more likely we will be motivated to eat healthier. It's almost a natural reaction.

How to Begin and Never Let It End

So once you've decided, "I want to do this," here are ways to get you started.

Don't Set Big Goals for Yourself

I believe that aggressive goal setting can sometimes be the worst thing you can do. It might be fine if you are already active and want to challenge yourself a little more, but if you are not currently getting enough exercise to be healthy, then you've got to work on just getting off the couch.

Getting Started

The biggest hurdle is getting started. If you're having trouble getting off the couch, try breaking down what you are trying to accomplish into smaller parts. For example, say you've committed yourself to walking for two miles and you're sitting on the couch thinking, "I don't want to do this." Take it one step at a time. Don't commit yourself to walking two miles. Instead try this:

Goal #1: Get off the couch.
Take a stretch, yawn and get up.

Goal #2: Get your shoes on, etc.

Now that you've put the task in motion,

Goal #3: Go outside (just to get some fresh air.
I can come back in if I want)

Goal #4: Walk around the block

Once you get started, the rest is easy. By the time you've made it around the block, walking two miles doesn't seem like such an effort. In fact, you might actually *want* to do it and you may be motivated to do more!

If you don't make the two miles today, don't give up. Try again tomorrow. Work towards your goal. Don't be disappointed because you didn't meet your goal. Congratulate yourself for doing more than you did before and go from there. By setting high or unrealistic expectations, you will most likely give up before you give yourself a chance.

Making the First Move

After a day of writing, my brain is fried and I could easily just lie on the couch and channel surf. On this particular day I had already been sneaking into the Valentine candy left on the counter. I felt tired, sluggish and did not look forward to doing anything except maybe eating some more. But, I don't like feeling tired and sluggish. I like to feel invigorated and energetic! I knew a neighborhood jog would perk me up but it was cold and very windy. I had only a half hour for myself so I had to make a decision. I called my neighbor. Maybe she would motivate me. "What, are you crazy? It's cold out there!" She was no help. I didn't want to do it. It was cold. I was tired.

Still unmotivated, I decided I would at least get ready to go. I dawdled around, stalling, and then finally put my headset on. With the music pumping, I finally decided to just step outside and see just how cold it really was! The wind slapped me in the face, the music was blaring and I started to run. And it felt great. I mean really great. Usually the worse I feel before, the better I feel during and afterwards. You know why? I really needed it!

My commitment was small. I was motivated only by my desire to feel better. I set no goals. I just got started.

Start small and go from there. If you belong to a gym, don't think, I have to do 30 minutes of cardio and 30 minutes of weight training. Just get in the car and drive.

When I was an aerobics instructor with Jazzercise, I had a student (an admitted couch potato) who fell in love with my class. She said to me one day, "You are such an inspiration. I never want to exercise, but all I have to do is get here and you do the rest for me. The music starts and before you know it an hour has passed and I feel great!"

Getting Better

While you shouldn't initially set big goals, once you've established regular exercise habits, increasing the duration and intensity of your activity will not only burn more calories, but will also decrease your risk of major health conditions and increase longevity. A Harvard study on exercise and longevity as reported in the *Journal of the American Medical Association* found that men who engaged in vigorous physical activity had a lower risk of death than men who engaged in lesser amounts of vigorous activity.

There are easy ways to increase your intensity and duration. Many people never realize their aerobic potential because they never allow their bodies to adjust to the aerobic curve. When you start an aerobic activity, your heart rate increases quickly, before your heart rate level has time to adjust. The hard part is getting from point A to point B. Any avid runner will tell you the first quarter-mile is the hardest because your heart rate goes from about 60 to about 130-150 beats per minute in a couple of minutes. That's when you feel most winded. That's when many people give up.

My best recommendation to anyone starting out is to allow your aerobic curve to increase slowly and then challenge yourself a little more. With walking or jogging, for example, start with a walk then increase your pace. If you listen to your body, it will tell you when you can go a little faster. When your heart rate gets a little higher, then you can try jogging or speed walking. Since your heart rate is already elevated from the walk, increasing it a little more at that point will be easier.

Even now I prefer to start a three-mile run with a 3-minute fast-paced walk. It makes the run more enjoyable. When I start with a walk, I never go through the huffing and puffing stage. I get into a good rhythm and increase it from there.

To increase intensity, during your walk practice short jogging or running sprints. For example, tell yourself, "I'm going to run from here to the third mailbox." When you successfully reach your goal start walking again. You'll discover your heart rate has elevated. Try it again a few minutes later and you will find the next sprint easier than the first because of your elevated heart rate. Do this consistently and you may find yourself a year later running in a 5K race!

Allow yourself to progress in activity by gradually increasing your aerobic curve and challenging yourself with short spurts of aerobic activity (some call this interval training). If you have already done your "exercise" for the day, don't pass up the opportunity to do more; take advantage of it. You'd be surprised at what you can do.

Don't Overthink It

It's easy to talk yourself out of anything you don't want to do. Put exercise on your list of things to do and just do it, instead of thinking about it. Is "I'm too busy" your excuse? Where is exercise on your busy list – after watching TV, playing on the Internet, talking endlessly on the phone? If you only have so much time in a day and exercise is a priority, you just do it so you can get on to the next thing. You don't have time to think about it.

Combine "not overthinking it" with taking small steps to meet goals and you can naturally motivate yourself. You tell yourself, "Okay, what's next on my list? Exercise. I better get ready." You run upstairs, put on your gym shoes and shorts and you're ready to go. Think of it as if you have to pick up the kids from soccer practice. You just do it.

Find Something Fun to Do

It's a shame that nowadays it's hard to participate in sports just for the fun of it. I remember on a nice evening my mom and dad would break out the old wooden tennis racquets and go to the high school and bat the ball around and have fun. It's hard to do that today. We have to have court time, a high-performance racquet, the right kind of shoes and a "rating." You don't go for a bike ride, you go "biking." People don't ask, "Do you like to play tennis?" They ask, "Do you *play* tennis?" If you say, "Yes," the next question is, "What's your rating?" When you say, "I don't have one," they are puzzled. You can't just like to play because it's fun.

Playing a sport has become so intimidating. You have to be good at it in order to be "worthy" of playing. You have to "take up" the game. This requires expensive lessons and specific time and date commitments. If you aren't naturally "athletic," the chance of you becoming a "worthy" player is even harder. Not only that, most instructors have higher expectations of their students and are less tolerant. So we just don't do it.

Having Fun I

Recently, a group of girlfriends and I challenged that trend when we went to Hilton Head together. Some of us were golfers, some were tennis players and some just came for well-deserved "R and R." One day we all went golfing. We spent nearly $100 for a round for golf but we had a blast. One of the girls had never picked up a club before.

We had the novice golfers play ahead of us. They goofed around, managed a few good shots and when they were frustrated or didn't keep pace, they picked up the ball and moved on to the next hole.

Golfing is a great game for women, but very intimidating. Most of us still fear the ball and the endless blanket of green. We think we have to keep score or finish every hole. But you know what? The golf police aren't going to arrest you if you don't! It's only a game. As long as you keep pace, don't worry about your game. Just have fun!

Having Fun II

Then we played tennis. I thought I could play pretty well. Boy was I wrong. Four of us reserved court time, showed up in our gym shorts, T-shirts, beat up sneakers and ancient tennis racquets (at least we did have new balls). Immediately we knew we were in trouble. Everyone else had at least $200 invested in their attire (and that doesn't include the racquet). You can't really hide from tennis like you can on the golf course. There we were smacking balls into the net, whiffing through the ball and knocking them over the fence. After a few minutes we forgot about all the dirty looks and started having a lot of fun. We actually managed a few good volleys which we all "high-fived" and made a big deal over.

Not Having Fun

While playing, we noticed a father coaching his daughter with intensity. She would look over from time to time and smile at us. Her father had walked away from her, disgusted at her performance. She looked sad. Then my friend yells over, "Hey! Want to play with us!" She didn't, but she did smile. We all thought she would have had more fun with us.

The Joy of Playing

Anyway, it is harder to just have fun exercising today. But see if you can explore some fun things to do without spending a lot of money. If you haven't experienced the joy of playing, you really are missing out on a lot. When was the last time you went biking? Swimming? Roller blading? When was the last time you tried a new sport? If you are unable to go outdoors, how about buying a funky dance video? You can have a lot of fun just doing stuff with your kids and you'll be a better parent for it.

Participating in 5k runs/walks for charity is great fun, especially when you get a group of people to do it. Some of us are afraid to try because we might be one of the last ones finished. Are we embarrassed? We shouldn't be. Coming in dead last in a 5K race is still better than not being able to do it at all. You are still the healthy minority. I've never gotten the impression that the first one to cross the finish line was treated with any more respect than the last one. Be proud of what you accomplished but most of all, have fun. Even with all my aerobic experience, I still come in at the bottom of any race I participate in. I do it to challenge myself, feel good and have fun!

Work on Your Self-Esteem

Don't avoid doing something fun because you're intimidated. This often happens when you are overweight and out of shape. When I taught aerobics, for example, overweight students would cluster in the back of the room like self-conscious wallflowers at the high school prom. I'd purposefully make sure I'd welcome them after class. I wanted them to feel comfortable. I wanted to reassure them that it was wonderful to have them in class. When they would comment on how bad they were, I would remind them that no one knows how to do the moves at first. Besides, everyone is too worried about themselves to pay attention to anyone else.

Richard Simmons' videos are great for the exercise challenged. It's comforting to see an overweight person on a video rather than a supermodel. And once they are comfortable in the privacy of their living room, exercising in public is easier.

The Only Thing Stopping You Is You

Low self-esteem can also prevent you from taking up a sport or any activity. Remember I told you that I received an award in high school for being the "worst" athlete? In gym, I couldn't run. I couldn't serve (or return) a volleyball. I feared a basketball and in field hockey I don't think I ever touched the ball with my stick, let alone make a goal. I didn't realize then that it wasn't due to my athletic inability, but my low self-esteem. When given an opportunity, I would succumb to my negative thoughts. "I can't do it" was always my motto instead of "You can do it!"

"I can't be like them. I'm not any good." Negative thoughts like these, coupled with the fact that I was out of shape, combined to produce pathetic results.

If you aren't confident in your ability, you are likely to fail. When I think about it, there were a few girls in my high school who were overweight but athletic. People gave them more respect. People didn't say they were "fat," they were "big." I wish I had realized that low self-esteem was the primary cause of my failures, not my weight. If I had any confidence I might not have had a weight problem in the first place. My self-labeled "inability" gave me an excuse to be fat.

Even today, I still plod along at a 10 mph jogging pace, I am mediocre at golf and I rarely win at tennis. I suspect my past history of "I can't" haunts me and prevents me from reaching my true potential. I'm no star athlete, but I get by and most importantly I have fun! I don't care what people think anymore. Life is too short.

Grab a Partner

Starting an activity with someone can be a great motivator and adds fun to your exercise. Whether it's walking, jogging, an aerobics class or a beginner golf or tennis lesson, a partner can increase the odds of sticking with it. I recently began jogging with a neighbor. I never did this before because I was always afraid I couldn't keep up. We go after work and it's a great stress reliever. Not only does the exercise make you feel better, but it's also an opportunity to vent with a captive audience about the frustrations of your day.

Ask your friends, relatives, coworkers or neighbors. Someone is bound to be looking for a motivator to help them get started.

Having a buddy to coax you along can help you stay on track. Many times I am feeling down and really don't want to do anything, let alone go outside when it's 40 degrees and take a walk. A quick phone call from my neighbor is all I need to get my butt in gear. Sometimes just the energy expended getting off the couch and hearing a friendly voice is enough to stimulate me. "I'll be up in 5 minutes," she says. And before you know it I'm on my second mile feeling great.

If your neighbor can't make it, try being your own buddy. If your buddy makes too many excuses and is interfering with your progress, look for another partner. The objective is to have someone that will help you succeed, not fail.

Stop Planning

I said this before. Stop saying, "I'm going to," or " I have to." There is no specific method – no right or wrong way. Exercise doesn't have to be timed, calculated or planned. Do anything and do it just for today. Just do more than you are doing now and keep it up. Do it every day and if you miss a day, don't quit. Do it the next day. Are you too busy to do the whole routine today? Then do 5 minutes.

I know so many people who smoked cigarettes and drank beer for the better part of their teens and 20's. They now run half-marathons and weight lift in their 40's. Do you think they planned to be like that? For a lot of them, just quitting smoking started the momentum. You are no different than anyone else and it's amazing what you can do. But if you keep planning, you can plan yourself to death.

Stop Excusing, Start Doing

Like eating healthier, you have to learn how to enjoy your life with exercise. Sitting on the couch, out of shape, you may say, I wouldn't enjoy any exercise. If you are suffering from low self-esteem you are probably thinking that you'd love to be like that, but you can't. That's someone else. Stop using your weight, athletic ability or your self-analysis as a justifiable excuse. Don't wait for some magic moment. One day you are going to find yourself too old, too fat or too sick. Then you'll realize the truth and think, "What the hell have I been doing all my life!" Don't have regrets. Even if you are 70, start today. There is so much more to living than working on a computer or staring at a television. Don't think of it as work. It's play! It's fun!

What Have We Learned?

- Moving your body is essential for your health
- The more you move, the better you will feel
- If you like to eat, you have to like to exercise
- Exercise shouldn't be grueling

STEP 8: Exercise for The NEW You

- Find something fun to do
- Move more throughout the day
- If you haven't used your body much today, it's probably not tired
- Don't overthink or set big goals
- You can do more than you think you can

Taking the First Steps

Each step is a goal:

Goal #1 Get off the couch
Goal #2 Get ready (shoes on, etc.)
Goal #3 Face your challenge
Goal #4 Begin your challenge

Once you begin, the rest is easy.

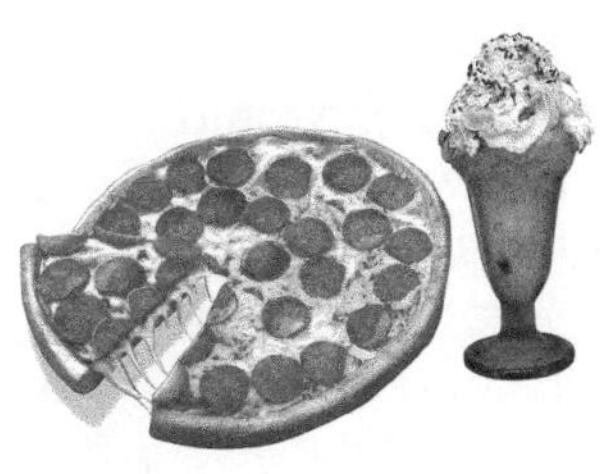

Chapter 16

STEP 9
Weight Training for The NEW You

Weight training is a small, but important component to successful long-term weight loss. Weight training increases metabolism, assists in adding and keeping bone density, protects bones from injury, helps keep and improve your figure and is mentally empowering. Weight training keeps your body young.

When I go to my basement gym, I always find it to be an empowering experience. I feel strong and beautiful and my head goes into a very good place. It's weight training and good nutrition (not low-calorie dieting) that keeps me from losing my figure. I feel young, much younger than 40-something, and I expect to continue to age gracefully.

Aesthetically Pleasing

Weight training is not about losing weight. Aesthetically, weight training allows you to improve your posture and reshape your body and makes the pounds you are – look better.

Many women who are unhappy with their post-baby figures try to fix the problem by losing weight. Most don't need to lose more weight; in fact, some are actually too thin and could benefit by gaining weight. Their problems usually include a paunchy tummy, bad posture and lack of muscle tone.

Instead of dieting, they would benefit more by lifting weights to improve their posture and muscle tone. If they gained a few pounds of muscle, their bodies would have more symmetry. With good nutrition, the body would work overtime feeding the new muscle and the fat in the belly might really start to melt away. If nothing else, better posture would make the tummy protrude less.

If you have big thighs and the rest of you isn't overweight, losing more weight might help you lose a little in your problem areas but you will also lose weight where you don't want to. Why is it that women with big thighs can diet themselves down to a triple A bra before they see any difference in their jeans! The problem with continued dieting is that you never improve your symmetry. You always look out of proportion.

Weight training helps you achieve better symmetry. If your hips are wider than your shoulders, you should work on developing your shoulders, chest and back along with minimizing your hip size. By broadening the shoulders and improving posture a woman can achieve better symmetry.

Getting Older, Getting Better

Weight training is most beneficial to aging women. I can't say enough about the health benefits of weight training for women. Osteoporosis is a debilitating and sometimes fatal disease that plagues mostly older women and is almost entirely preventable.

The National Institute on Aging says, "Osteoporosis is preventable. A diet that is rich in calcium and vitamin D and a lifestyle that includes regular weight-bearing exercises are the best ways to prevent osteoporosis."

As we get older, the loss of muscle and the depletion of calcium make our bones brittle and more vulnerable to breakage.

By weight training you can maintain your muscle and your strength well into your golden years. God willing, I plan to be walking a golf course and hauling mulch for my garden when I'm 80.

If You Don't Use It, You Lose It

Aesthetically, weight training is the best defense against the effects of aging. As we age, we lose muscle tone and we lose our shape.

Deborah L. Mullen, CSCS, agrees. "Inactive adults lose around one-half pound of muscle per year, or 5 pounds per decade. If you take in more calories then you burn, the extra calories get stored as fat. Fat is less dense then muscle – a pound of fat takes up more room than a pound of muscle. This means that as you lose muscle and gain fat, your weight might remain the same over the years, but your waistline will continue to expand!"

Many women try to lose weight in an effort to regain their lost figure. For aging women, while the result might be less weight on the scale, the downside is their skin sags and they end up looking older. As long as I keep weight training and continue to eat right and exercise, I will be able to keep my figure. I care more about my shape than the scale. If I lose weight, my skin starts sagging and while I may wear a smaller pant size, I look older. At 42, I think I'd rather look younger than be a size 4.

Along with keeping my figure young, by maintaining muscle I can eat like a younger person too! A Tufts University study found that people who strength-trained for three months on a regular basis added 3 pounds of muscle. And the subjects found they had to eat 15 percent more calories just to maintain their body weight.

Myths and Misconceptions

Weight training is catching on, but many still resist it. Women have fears they will get big and muscular. Some are intimidated by it; many people don't have the right equipment. Another problem is people get injured because they don't know how to do it. Men, especially, don't look for help and insist on lifting way too much weight, too soon. They execute a movement incorrectly and they end up on the chiropractor's table. Here are some common excuses for not weight training.

I'll Get Too Muscular

I lift fairly heavy weights, but have no fears of getting too muscular. Some women are afraid they will get big and bulky. They see steroid "she-men" and think that's what's going to happen to them.

While it is rare for women to have enough testosterone to develop excessive muscle mass, if you don't also incorporate good nutrition and exercise with weight training, you could end up with muscle hiding under fat.

I remember briefly training a woman who had lost 30 pounds on Weight Watchers. She wasn't overweight, but what extra weight she had was in her thighs. She was exercising frequently – taking aerobic classes and walking three miles a few times a week – while staying on the Weight Watchers food program.

I began to notice that while her legs were still big, she was looking too thin in the face and upper body. She was also sick a lot. I suspected she probably wasn't eating enough and feared she might become anorexic. I suggested weight training might help her more than losing more weight. She reluctantly agreed, because she didn't want to become muscular.

During our first session I handed her a 3-pound weight and showed her how to perform a simple one-arm row exercise for her back. She started the movement, stopped, looked at me and said, "Are you sure it's all right, I won't get big muscles?" It was our first and last session. The woman had the willpower and desire, but couldn't get over the fear.

I'll Gain Weight

Many women quit weight training because they don't lose weight. We are so obsessed with the scale. It is a fact that if you build more muscle you might gain weight especially if you aren't losing body fat in the process. Muscle weighs more than fat. The goal is to build muscle and lose fat. Building muscle can increase your metabolism, but you still need to practice good nutrition and regular cardiovascular conditioning. It's a *combination* of these components that creates unbelievable long-term results.

My personal story substantiates this. I lost weight about 9 years ago. I went from 155 to 135 pounds. I wasn't on a specific diet, but I had started a new job after my last baby and I was renewed and motivated. I gave up Dunkin Donuts and was "doing" power lunches. After buying a new wardrobe of sleek fitting size 6 business suits, the novelty wore off and the weight started creeping up. The skirts were tight around the thighs and would ride up when I walked and stay up after I sat down.

I kept trying to lose the weight to no avail. I was doomed. It was just a matter of time before I went back to my old weight.

After reading an article in *Muscle and Fitness* on female fitness competitors and their diet and training habits I decided to start weight training again. This time I also changed my diet to include more protein, fruits, vegetables and whole grains. I also started lifting heavier weights.

I liked lifting weights. It made me feel strong and energized. There was only one problem. I was still gaining weight. My weight had shot up 10 pounds and I thought, "This isn't working!"

Yet, I was still able to get into my size 6 clothes. In fact, they started to fit better. They weren't loose, but they fit me differently. They were snug around the butt, but not at the thighs (the saddlebags). They didn't ride up anymore. I also noticed my posture had improved. I stood taller and my stomach appeared flatter. My body started getting curves in all the right places.

Even with the positive visual change, I was reluctant to accept the weight gain. There were times I would crash diet or stop lifting so I could lose weight. It just didn't make sense to me that I could weigh almost 150 pounds and be a size 6. The same weight I was when I wore a size 12.

Eventually the positive effects of weight training were being reported. Better educated, I recognize now that until I can't get into my clothes, I don't care what the scale says.

My sister, who I see only once every few years, once said to me, "Where did you get that body! You have ankles! You have shoulders! Your stomach is so flat! Your figure is completely different!"

I believe the weight training is why many people assume I was an athlete in high school. I'm not thin, but I look athletic – healthy. I actually prefer looking athletic over looking thin.

I Don't Know How

Many people don't weight train because they don't know how. We might be motivated to give it a try but sometimes it's easier said than done. Some people quit after a bad experience of confusion or embarrassment. They might injure themselves or experience abnormal discomfort because they aren't doing the movement correctly.

The most common method for a beginner is to join a gym and use the weight machines. Gyms typically require a club trainer to instruct you on the proper use of the machines. The "instruction" usually consists of a 20-minute run through of every piece of equipment and how it works. Then you are on your own.

While the equipment is relatively easy to operate, it's confusing at first. Each piece of equipment has a different use and method of operation. So the next time you come to the gym you don't remember what the trainer told you. The trainers in the gym are there to help you, but you have to get their attention and some of us are embarrassed to ask for help. That experience alone is enough to get most people to give it up.

Knowing how a machine works and knowing how to perform a movement are two completely different things. Whether using a machine or free weights, if you aren't performing the movement correctly, you are more susceptible to injury and you won't get the best results for the time spent.

Gyms offer personal trainers to help you learn the proper technique, but to maximize your experience, you really need to get individualized help. That means a separate, and sometimes expensive fee.

If you can afford it, I think the best and fastest way to learn proper weight training technique is to hire a personal trainer for about two months, preferably in your home. Buy a few starter weights and have your trainer personally teach you the proper form. Make doubly sure you learn which muscle groups you exercise with each movement. I know so many people who weight train for months and don't even know what muscle they are supposed to be working with the varied exercises.

The Easiest Way to Learn

I didn't learn how to weight train from a gym. I educated myself at home. I bought some inexpensive dumbbells, and read as much as I could about the subject. I taped ESPN shows that educated people on body sculpting. Truthfully, I learned more from my own research than I did studying for my personal training certification. If you don't have money to invest, educating yourself at home is cheap and just as educational.

Group classes are also good, inexpensive options. Most aerobic classes include a 15 minute strength training/stretching session. Many, like Jazzercise and most YMCA's, offer both low and high impact classes. You're sure to find one that suits your ability. Yoga and Pilates are both good strength-training options as well.

Keeping It Up

Once you know the fundamentals, you can advance at your own pace. You can invest more money in equipment or join a gym. If you join a gym, I recommend having at least a few dumbbells at home in case your life gets too busy and you haven't the time to get there.

I use both. I weight train about three times a week, but often I prefer to weight train at home. I like the variety. A quick 20-minute session a few times a week at home is a lot easier than a two-hour gym commitment. And with an in home gym I can't use "I don't have time to get to the gym" as an excuse.

People assume you need fancy equipment in order for strength training to work but that's not the case. I can do a full body weight training routine with only a few sets of dumbbells. The results are just as good if not better than if I used all the machine weights at the gym. High tech gyms are great, but they are overrated. The most important thing is safety first. Learn how to do it, don't overdo it and listen to your body. Focus on the movements and the muscle you are working

I'm Too Self-Conscious

Learning how to weight train at a gym can be intimidating. This is especially true if serious weight lifters dominate the training room. I can't give you a lesson in self-confidence. I suffered with this too. As I got older, though, I became wiser.

You have just as much right to be there as anyone. You paid your dues just like they did. Everyone starts somewhere. In reality, most weight lifters are more than happy to make room for you and most like to be asked for help. If they don't, they are self-absorbed. That's their problem, not yours.

Weight lifting is also narcissistic. For maximum results you need to focus on your muscle when performing the movement. That means focusing on yourself and your body.

Many of us are resistant to that kind of intense self-examination. However, if you can get past the first doubting glances, you will find that watching your muscles move (even if they are under a layer of fat) is very empowering. You get in touch with your body and your self.

I recommend that you expose as much of your muscle as possible during weight training. Try not to wear baggy T-shirts and big gym pants. Most people assume weight lifters who wear skimpy clothes are show-offs. While there are those that want to show off their stuff, most expose their bodies to monitor their progress and to be more focused on the muscle they are training. I have a much better workout if I watch my body in the mirror than if I stared at a wall in a T-shirt.

By watching yourself you develop a mind/body connection. Remember when I talked about ignoring your body by covering it up. By mentally connecting your mind with your body you learn to identify with and appreciate your body. I call it the mind/body connection. The mind/body connection is very good for the spirit and is motivating.

If you are reluctant to go to the gym, start out at home. Expose your curves and use a mirror. "Ugh," you say? Trust me. No matter how you look at the start, if you stick with it, a friendly mirror will help you meet your goals.

Pick Up a Weight, Pick Up Good Habits

The best thing about weight training is you don't have to be athletic or have cardiovascular stamina to do it. I know of many people who started their journey to good health by picking up a weight. Anyone can do it. The empowering experience then spills over into other healthy behaviors.

The benefit of weight training outweighs the time invested in learning how to do it. While typically considered anaerobic, weight training has cardiovascular benefits. It has an advantage over aerobic activity because you don't have to be athletic to do it. You don't have to join a gym to get started and the initial investment is small.

Eating less will help you lose weight. Weight lifting will give you a shapelier and healthier body. Trust me. Get out the weights; you'll thank yourself for it.

What Have We Learned?

- Weight training can help prevent osteoporosis
- Muscle weighs more than fat
- Muscle needs more fuel (food) than fat
- Inactive adults lose about one half pound of muscle every year – weight training slows the process
- Weight training can help you keep or improve your figure
- You don't have to have athletic ability or stamina to weight train

How to Get Started

- Join a gym, hire a personal trainer or buy a set of dumbbells

STEP 9: Weight Training for The NEW You

- Don't let a trainer blindly lead you
- Get educated. Learn your muscle groups and the applicable exercises
- Safety first. Don't overdo it
- Practice the mind/body connection

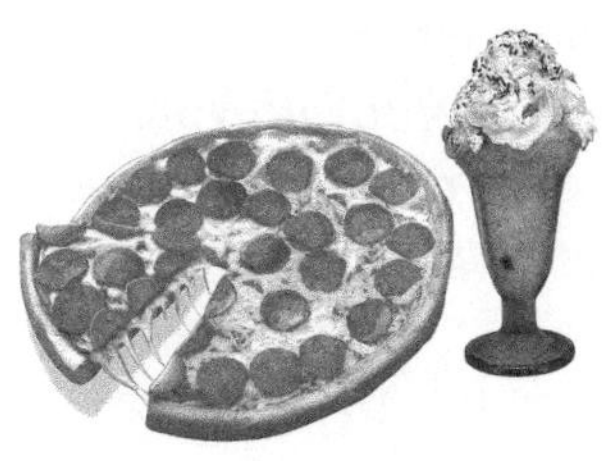

Chapter 17

Final Plans for a Fabulous Future

At the beginning of this book, I vented my anger towards the destruction, deceits, lies and insanity of the American dieting marketplace. I concluded that the result of this decade of disillusionment is we've become a society obsessed with food. And the harder we try to lose weight, it seems, the more difficult it becomes. The more we buy, the more bizarre the marketers' shenanigans become to find a way – any way – to sell their bill of goods.

Accept reality. There are no magic plans or silver bullets that will make you suddenly thin. The "magic" lies within you.

I made a comparison of our diet problems to pieces of a puzzle. Without all the pieces, the puzzle isn't complete. I hope the 9 Steps to The NEW You program provided the pieces to your puzzle so you now have the tools to create your own your "magic" answer.

Creating the "Magic"

Discovering *your* answer is a process. What pieces do you need to put your puzzle together? You need to analyze the way you think, listen and behave with regards to food, your expectations and how you choose to live.

To implement the path to success, you might want to keep a journal and while you go through the steps keep track of the thoughts, actions and behaviors that you need to improve. Chart your food consumption, how much you move, your bad habits and your emotions. Find out your real problem and take action.

Most importantly, keep your journal honest. To thine own self be true. It takes self-discovery and time. Be honest, find your problem(s), take action and, before you know it, you will become The NEW You.

Are you ready to tackle the process and truthfully analyze and identify the reason(s) you are overweight? Once you know why you are overweight, you can map out a plan to solve your weight problem. Let's review the pieces of the puzzle. Decide what pieces you need to use in order to solve your problem and develop your own path to success – to The NEW You!

Reality Check – A New Way of Thinking

I suggested that you take a good, hard look at the way you view yourself and your relationship with food. Our environment may negatively affect how you feel about yourself and your relationship with food. You might be relying on high-calorie, convenient foods and believe it's out of your control. Maybe you have lost sight of reality when it comes to your expectations of how your body can look and you feel weak, powerless and unworthy.

Maybe you are confused about what you are supposed to eat. You've been bombarded with so many theories it's no wonder you might be obsessed with food. Do you feel guilty eating? Do you analyze everything you eat? Do you really enjoy eating anymore?

Do you feel the situation is hopeless? If so, you may have gone into denial about what you eat and how much you eat. You might selectively remember what and how much you really eat. Whether it's not recognizing a serving size, not counting a handful of crackers or chipping away at the apple pie resulting in two unacknowledged pieces – if you can't admit the actions, you can't do anything about them.

You might choose to blame or make excuses for your inability to lose weight. Blaming takes the responsibility off of ourselves by blaming something else for our inability to lose weight. "I'm fat, but it's not my fault!"

If you are blaming, excusing or denying, then you need to be honest with yourself. Are you ready to come clean? Are you ready to admit what you really eat and that maybe you are to blame?

Accepting Realities

We are told we can be aesthetically perfect and do it in six weeks. You have to ditch that fantasy and accept reality. Believing fantasies portrayed by the media and the diet industry makes us feel hopeless. We give up because our goals are unrealistic. Understand and accept these realities:

- Your body is unique. You can only achieve your potential, not someone else's.
- It takes a long time to lose weight – real weight. And that means you must like the changes to achieve long term success. You can only punish yourself with a diet for so long. Take your time and enjoy the ride.
- You can't change your lifestyle overnight. Even small improvements can benefit your health significantly. Change gradually and adapt to your new lifestyle.
- Reevaluate your goals as they are achieved.
- Change will not happen unless you apply the basic principles of losing weight. Calories in/calories out. That's the only way it works.
- Measure success by how you feel, not how you look.

If you are living in a fantasy about what you can achieve, you are setting yourself up for failure. Do you understand and accept the realities of your potential, how you lose weight and how you measure success? With your new way of thinking you will be able to reach obtainable, life changing goals.

Accepting Change

Before you attempt change, you have to want to change, be convinced you can change and make a firm decision to change. You can't just want to be thin – you have to live like a thin person. If you aren't ready to make that commitment, you needn't bother trying to implement the actions that produce change. You will inevitably fail.

A New Way of Listening

If you listen to your body's signals, it will tell you what it wants and how much it wants. The problem is you may not be listening.

You don't have to give up any food you enjoy, but you have to practice moderation. Before you overindulge, think about how you will feel if you eat more. Is it really going to taste good? Are the 2-minute pleasures of eating worth the two hours of pain – feeling stuffed and mad at yourself?

Think about what you want to eat and don't eat anything you really don't want. Save your indulgences for foods you really enjoy. If you don't want it, don't put it in your mouth.

The important factors are thinking before you act and being accountable for what you eat. Take a moment to consider what you are eating, how much you are eating and why you are eating it.

Listening to your body is easier than you think. Are you ready to practice your listening skills? It doesn't happen overnight, but the results in both weight loss and heightened food enjoyment are worth the effort.

Bad Habits Are Bad News

Recognize and acknowledge the bad habits that contribute to your weight problem. Are you guilty of being an overeater, an emotional eater or a mindless eater? Do you eat on the run? Identify your bad habits and work towards minimizing the damage caused by your unsavory actions. Bad habits are hard to break, so don't expect to succeed overnight. In fact don't expect to break them entirely. Work on damage control. Recognize what you are doing and take action to minimize the damage.

A New Way of Behaving – The NEW You

Once you've accepted reality and adopted new ways of thinking and listening, you're ready to take on the challenges of the actual *doing*. That means eating and exercising to your full potential. Are you ready for that change? Do you accept the reality that you are going to have to eat better, get regular exercise and strength train for the rest of your life?

Nutrition, Exercise and Weight Training – it sounds overwhelming. But it's not. To the contrary, the three components together make the process of change easier. They feed off each other.

One healthy habit easily leads to more healthy habits. Picking up a weight can be the stimulus needed for confidence. The aerobics class you took after work got you out of the dumps and helped you resist methodical, emotional eating. Choosing the healthier entrée gave you the energy to take a walk. The pound of muscle you gained allowed you to eat an extra cookie a day without repercussion.

Learn to eat and enjoy *real* food again. Get educated on the basic principles of nutrition. Don't be duped by false claims and misleading information.

Take advantage of every opportunity to move your body. Strengthen your body both inside and out through weight training. Make it a hobby.

Seize the Day

The time to start is now because *every* day is the day. Do it every day. Do what? Pay attention to what you eat. Work daily exercise into your life. Those two bites of whatever you ate today you didn't even want can make a difference. Playing kickball with your kids for 10 minutes instead of saying, "Not right now, Mommy's tired," can be the trigger for a lifetime of change. Don't go through life saying, "I've got to start dieting" or "I've got to start exercising." Stop planning, failing and blaming – just do it!

My Final Send-Off

It took me years, but I found and followed my path to success. I discovered I didn't have one weight issue, but a multitude of issues. A lot of little problems, that, when combined, caused a big problem in how I viewed food and myself. I realize now my problem wasn't about losing weight. It was about freeing myself of my obsessive behaviors. My fear of food, my desire to be aesthetically perfect, my denial and bad habits. Allowing food and the mirror to dictate whether I was good or bad, weak or strong, worthy or not worthy. I set myself free by believing and behaving like someone I thought I could never be.

Today I *am* the person I thought I could never be. I trust myself with food. I enjoy food – all food – more than ever. I am happy with my imperfect body. I don't waste time thinking about what's "good" or "bad," I just listen to my body and give it what it wants – what it *really* wants. I don't work out – I play. I love to play.

I eat healthy and exercise because it makes me feel good. I want to be the best I can be, not for someone else's approval, but because my life is happier because of it.

Before you read this book, you might not have been aware of

the negative behaviors that are the real cause of your weight problems. The solution, you thought, was in finding a diet that would make you lose weight. Book after book, product after product you tried – and failed. I hope you will now stop looking and start evaluating. Find your real problem(s) and then embrace the journey to find your answer.

Don't believe that because you have a weight problem you are different from others and powerless to change. Don't conclude that you aren't an exercise person or you are a food addict or that eating healthy is a sacrifice. Believe that you can be a person without weight issues – a person who enjoys activity, prefers to be a healthy eater and is happy with their body.

If you can eliminate the obstacles that prevent you from losing weight – the negative thoughts, the negative way you listen to your body's needs and your negative behaviors – your problem will be solved forever.

Eat healthy, get regular exercise and learn to enjoy food again – all foods: even pizza and ice cream.

I wish for you a healthier, happier life.

After Word

I've tried to address all of the problems you might have with food, weight and how you feel about yourself. If, after reading this book, you still can't find your answer or have problems implementing your answer, please contact me.

My goal is to help everyone with their weight issues. The more I find out about how and why people eat, the better educated I am to help others solve their problems.

Help me out, won't you? Visit my website at www.pizzaandicecreamdiet.com and we can help you find *your* answer.